This book is a breath of fresh air! Parijat has somehow managed to explore the often dark and anxiety-producing topic of high-risk pregnancy in a positive and even joyful manner. She knows what it's like to experience a high-risk pregnancy, and is deeply familiar with the abundant research on the effects of stress during pregnancy. Through these pages, she weaves her personal experiences and professional knowledge in a seamless and easy-to-read manner, that makes apparent why she's rightfully earned the title of high-risk pregnancy expert. This book is a required, confidence-building and health-supporting read for anyone facing a stress-filled pregnancy.

ADRIANA LOZADA
Maternity expert and host of the Birthful podcast

Parijat Deshpande has created a "must read" for all women in a high-risk pregnancy. The title says it all: *Pregnancy Brain: A Mind-Body Approach to Reducing Stress During Your High-Risk Pregnancy*. Nothing could be more important for both you and your baby. By gently sharing her personal journey, Parijat removes the fears of the Unknown. *Pregnancy Brain* read like a kitchen table conversation with a friend. This beautifully written book delivers a critically important message.

SUSAN ANDREWS PhD
Clinical Neuropsychologist

A story of hope, inspiration, and raw emotion with a healthy dose of practical wisdom for those dealing with the ins and outs of a difficult pregnancy. Get your hands on this book if you want to know that somebody gets you and—even better—can help you move yourself through, often unspeakable, emotional and physical pain.

MARIA T. ROTHENBURGER, PhD
Fertility Coach and Therapist

Pregnancy Brain is a groundbreaking book that's going to change the way expecting moms and their providers view stress management, mental health, and self care. Parijat empowers mothers to take an active role in reducing their risk of complications and preterm birth, all by accessing the power of their mind. Best of all, it's written in a way that makes you want to keep reading until you get to the end.

LILY NICHOLS, RDN, CDE
Bestselling author of Real Food for Pregnancy and Real Food for Gestational Diabetes
lilynicholsRDN.com

As I read this book, I got so excited to finally see this information laid out in an easily digestible, conversational, non-alarmist manner. Not only is this book great for pregnancy, it's great information for overall mental health, whether or not you're pregnant. So many books on topics such as these may hold fascinating information with an incredibly boring presentation. Not this book! I plan on sharing this book with all my clients, especially those in high risk pregnancies. Thank you so much for this valuable resource!

LORI LYNN TUCKER,
Doula at lorilynntuckerdoula.com
Rogers, Arkansas

This book is the best combination of personal storytelling, engaging information, real education and science. I believe the way that Parijat has woven together story with science is such an effective way to support women and families in the reproductive period. Many people will both learn about their bodies and feel truly seen throughout this book. This is such an empowering and real contribution to reproductive health.

KATAYUNE KAENI, PSY.D.
Psychologist in Perinatal Mental Health, Mom & Mind Podcast
www.momandmind.com

pregnancy brain.

*A Mind-Body Approach to
Stress Management During a
High-Risk Pregnancy*

Parijat Deshpande, MS

ISBN (Paperback): 978-1-7324197-0-4
ISBN (Ebook): 978-1-7324197-1-1

Where case studies and professionals appear, real names, professions, locations, and other biographical details have been changed to preserve their privacy and anonymity.

The author of this book does not dispense medical or psychological advice or prescribe the use of any technique as a form of treatment for physical, emotional or medical problems without the advice of a licensed physician or medical professional or licensed mental health provider, either directly or indirectly. This book is for general informational purposes only and is not a substitute for medical or psychological attention, treatment, examination, advice, or diagnosis from a licensed medical or mental health practitioner.

In the event you use any of the information in this book for yourself, the author and the publisher assume no responsibility for your actions.

Library of Congress Control Number: 2018947004

Cover Design by: Angela Greaser, AllTheOps.com
Layout and interior design by: Melinda Martin, MartinPublishingServices.com

For Vihaan

*May your life continue to be filled
with miracles that take your breath away.*

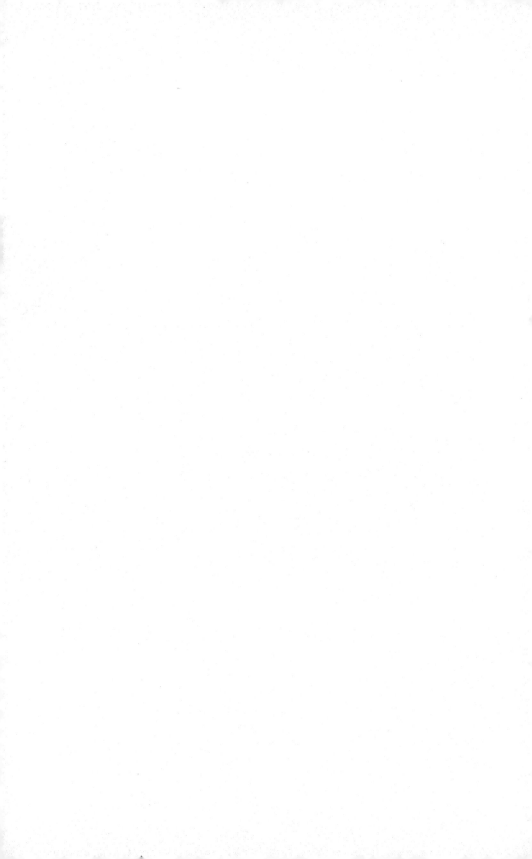

CONTENTS

INTRODUCTION

Creating Miracles

Impossible situations can become possible miracles.

—Robert H. Schuller

When I was about 12 years old, my dad clipped out an article from a newspaper, put it on our refrigerator, and told my brother and me, "This is why we need to be more positive in life."

It was the story of a man who had suffered a massive heart attack. His doctors had given him a poor prognosis, but the man didn't accept the bleak future painted for him. Since he had nothing to lose, he decided to take matters into his own hands. You've surely heard the phrase "Laughter is the best medicine." He took that old adage to heart and committed to laughing every single day—not just chuckling or giggling, but doing whatever it took to get those deep belly laughs.

The news article shared that his serious heart condition improved without explanation by his medical team, and he was discharged from the hospital, something his physicians told him would likely not happen.

I was shocked, curious, and mesmerized.

What had happened to him? How had he beaten the awful prognosis the doctors were sure was his future? If he could do it, could others?

Did laughter cure this man in the news story of his heart disease? No. Proponents of laughter therapy will be the first to tell you that laughter is not a cure-all solution. However, what scientists have found repeatedly is that interventions like laughter are so much more powerful than being simply mood-enhancing techniques. They create neurological, immunological, and cellular changes in your body that allow for healing to occur.[1]

For years, I have thought of that news article and the man who beat the odds. My dad had intended for this article to show us the importance of being more optimistic, happy people instead of the broody teens we were becoming, but what it did for me was far more profound than that.

It planted a seed in my brain that over the years would sprout and grow into a vastly huge idea. One that I would get to test myself during several medical crises in my life. One that would challenge people's notions of what health really means.

That idea is that we have the power to create our own medical miracles by influencing our health. This power comes from our ability to manage our physical, emotional, relational, and environmental stress effectively because our body's systems are all interconnected and depend on, as well as influence, each other for optimal physical health and functioning.

It's an idea contrary to what the field of medicine tells us. To be honest, it took me a long time to speak out publicly about this because it challenges so many deeply held beliefs about what our bodies can and cannot do, what *we* can and cannot do, and what *doctors* can and cannot do in the face of health complications, especially during pregnancy.

Just as a plant blossoms with leaves, sometimes outgrowing the pot in which it was originally potted, so grew this idea until I couldn't ignore it anymore.

Clearly, I wasn't the first to consider the possibility that lifestyle changes and stress management were important—critical—to achieving optimal health and wellness. The mind-body connection has been addressed by the medical field, neuroscientists, and health advocates for nearly a century.

So when I began my research into stress management and lifestyle medicine to improve pregnancy outcomes, imagine my surprise when I heard crickets. I only found a handful of articles in mainstream media sharing this message. It was as if the role of stress during pregnancy was an afterthought to medical professionals and women alike. There was a feeling that the impact of stress on pregnancy was being hidden behind a curtain that's best not to open. It's safe to say most of us have a vague understanding that stress is bad for health, but women do not regularly, if at all, receive information about the details of how it impacts health specifically during pregnancy.

Once I opened my private practice offering stress-management health consultations for pregnant women, I was inundated with emails from women sharing their stories of stress during pregnancy. I received dozens upon dozens of emails from women recounting their stories of loss, convinced their stress played a role. Emails from women who raised their concerns with their obstetricians about how anxiety was impacting their pregnancy or growing baby, only to be brushed off. Emails from women who asked for referrals for mental health providers, to not be seen for months due to long waitlists and insurance blocks. These were women desperate for answers to confirm what their gut was telling them and tools for how to prevent a similar experience in future pregnancies.

This infuriated me. Why were women not receiving the support and information they need to understand how stress negatively impacts pregnancy and how effective stress management can create positive changes in a pregnancy? There *had* to be literature out there showing a connection between stress, pregnancy complications, and preterm delivery. There also had to be literature out there showing the connection between effective stress *management* and positive pregnancy outcomes.[2]

If there is evidence that stage-four cancer can go into remission,[3] chronic illness can be cured,[4] and heart disease can be reversed[5] because of the impact of the mind-body connection, why can't we expect that effective stress management can improve the health of a high-risk pregnancy and reduce the risk of preterm delivery?

My search deepened and became more fervent. I delved deep into the research. *Somebody had to know about this.* What I found, shocked me and sent me down a rabbit hole that led me to a gold mine. People weren't just talking about it. There has been more than 70 years of research, literature, and science documenting the dramatic mind-body connection between stress and fertility, pregnancy, prenatal complications, and preterm delivery.

Reading the works of professionals in the field of mind-body science such as Dr. Herbert Benson, Dr. Bruce Lipton, Dr. Norman Cousins, and Dr. Lissa Rankin took my breath away. Expanding my research into the works of pioneers in perinatal psychology and wellness such as Dr. Chris Dunkel-Schetter, Dr. Christine Guardino, Dr. Thomas O'Connor, and Dr. Susan Andrews lit a fire under me. Devouring the empirical data of the impact of stress specifically on pregnancy by leading high-risk obstetricians and psychoneuroimmunology experts Dr. Calvin Hobel, Dr. Patik Wadhwa, and Dr. Mary Coussons-Read confirmed the enormity of the connection between stress and pregnancy health.

It was like opening up the hall closet you never let anyone near, because the minute the door swings wide, everything falls out. Well, let me tell you, everything fell out and I found myself buried under a pile of evidence-based research showing the tremendous impact that stress has on pregnancy and preterm delivery.[6] The connection is *so* major, *so* robust, and *so* profound that it impacts families for generations.

Researchers, scientists, and clinicians have spent decades upon decades doing this work and have found find empirical evidence—scientific proof—that your mental state causes physiological changes in the body that affect pregnancy and the growing fetus.

It is mind-blowing how it works.

To carry a healthy pregnancy, changes to your hormones, your nervous system, and your immune system are necessary. Nature has ensured that during pregnancy, the shifts in each of these body systems are kept in delicate balance—all to help you have a healthy pregnancy and carry a baby to term.

The immune system is suppressed so your body doesn't reject the foreign tissue (your baby) but not so suppressed that you are too sick to be able to carry the baby to term. The endocrine system increases production of certain hormones to levels higher than any other time in your life to help you stay pregnant without being so high that they throw other hormones completely out of whack. Your nervous system is kept in perfect balance, secreting stress hormones in a carefully titrated manner to help you stay pregnant, help your baby grow and thrive, and then prepare you for labor and delivery.

It's a perfectly choreographed dance among all three major biological systems that's naturally built into your body to help you have a healthy pregnancy and deliver a healthy baby. However, physical, emotional, relational, and environmental stress has been shown to create an imbalance among these three body systems, which can profoundly impact pregnancy health. It's like a domino tilted just a bit too much that halts the pattern, preventing the pattern from falling in one swift motion.

Through my work, I recognized that it is not the cognitive or emotional aspects of stress, but the physical symptoms that are most important to address during a high-risk pregnancy. The cognitive and emotional experiences, though important, are not nearly as telling about how much stress is impacting your pregnancy as are the physical symptoms, such as high blood pressure, elevated blood glucose levels, preterm contractions, aches and pains, insomnia. The biggest giveaway is the existence of pregnancy complications that are dependent on the delicate balance of the three body systems, such as preeclampsia, preterm labor, gestational diabetes, intrauterine growth restriction (IUGR), chorioamnionitis, placental abruption, and shortening of the cervix, among others.[7]

Here's how this works.

You've surely had the experience of getting ready to give a presentation or have a difficult conversation when all of a sudden you start to feel changes in your body.

Headaches.
Dry mouth.
Sweaty hands.
Muscle pains.
Digestive problems.
Insomnia.
Heart palpitations.
Vomiting.
Nausea.

Sound familiar?

You're anxious. You're worried. You're nervous. Those thoughts and those feelings trigger a stress response in your body, activating a part of your nervous system getting you ready to fight or run. This physiological stress response is exactly the same whether you're being chased by a grizzly bear, fighting with your partner, or waiting for tests results during your pregnancy.[8]

Consciously, you know that you're not being chased by a grizzly bear, but the most primitive part of your brain—the lizard brain, as it's so affectionately called—which sits right above the brainstem above your spine, has no idea of the difference.

It perceives a threat (either an actual bear or repetitive thoughts about how you're not good enough for the promotion or worry about a test result that will tell you something's wrong with the baby). It then triggers a part of your brain called the hypothalamus (part of the hypothalamic-pituitary-adrenocortical axis, or the HPA axis) that fires up your sympathetic nervous system, and you're in fight or flight mode. Your stress response is on.

It's like a biological workflow that happens every single time you feel scared, uncertain, nervous, anxious, or helpless, no matter the trigger. The lizard brain identifies a problem, interprets it as a safety issue like being chased by a grizzly bear, and prepares your body to fight or run.

Lizard brain. Grizzly bear. Run.

When the stress response is activated, the delicate balance among the endocrine, immune, and nervous systems is disrupted. Blood moves from your core to your arms and legs, preparing you to run to safety. Your heart rate and breathing rate increase, pumping your body to prepare for battle or running away (leaving you feeling hot and sweaty). Digestion slows down (hence the stomachaches before your doctor's appointment). Your mouth goes dry. You feel wide awake and alert (explaining the insomnia for the few nights before family comes into town). Reproductive function declines because—let's face it—having babies is a luxury if your brain thinks you're under attack.[9]

When the stress response is on, there is an increase of inflammation in your body, a dampening of your immune system, which increases your risk of getting sick or contracting and infection,[10] and reduces your ability to heal. Additionally, the stress response promotes production of stress hormones, one of which is called the corticotropin-releasing hormone (CRH). CRH is a hormone that's essential for starting labor at term.[11] When stress levels reach a particular threshold, early in the pregnancy, enough of that hormone accumulates labor begins prematurely.[12]

High levels of stress hormones in the body have also been connected with preeclampsia,[13] diminished blood flow to the baby, small for gestational age babies, gestational diabetes, shortening cervix, and rupture of the amniotic sac preterm, preterm contractions,[14] preterm labor,[15] as well as placental abruption.[16]

When stress hormones course through your body, biological changes happen almost instantaneously. The only goal your brain and body have is to get away from the threat. Everything else is deprioritized by shifts in the immune, endocrine, and neurological systems. During pregnancy, those shifts, if present for long enough, set the stage for certain pregnancy complications.

However, activation of the stress response is not actually the problem. Our bodies are designed to be able to handle high stress in short bursts, even during pregnancy. The problem arises when your body doesn't have a chance to reset after the stress response to recover, repair, and regain that balance among the three body systems.

Our bodies have a built-in repair system that activates to fix all of the damage this stress response creates in your body. This relaxation system, called the relaxation response by cardiologist Dr. Herbert Benson in the 1970s, is an "inducible, physiological state" that has a whole-body effect to recover from periods of physical, emotional or situational stress.[17] This relaxation response restores proper digestion and deep breathing. It helps you go to sleep and wake feeling rested. Blood pressure declines. Reproductive function is restored. Blood oxygen levels rise. Smooth muscles relax. Physical pain diminishes. High-quality sleep is restored. Insulin levels stabilize. Blood flow optimizes. Proper immune function returns. Inflammation decreases. Repair of cellular damage begins.[18]

The best part is, it's a system that you can turn on at any time.

A client of mine who experienced this for the first time during a session together told me it felt like being relaxed and energized at the same time. That's exactly the goal of the this self-repair mechanism. When this relaxation system is turned on, your body is able to repair the damage that stress caused and heal from whatever health condition you're experiencing because balance is restored among the three systems, a balance that is impossible to have when you are experiencing the hormonal, neurological, and immune effects of stress.

Sometimes that healing leads to spontaneous cures and sometimes the healing occurs just enough to pull you out of the danger zone.[19] It creates a sense of physical relaxation that allows your body to get pregnant[20] and have a healthy pregnancy. It sets the stage for medical miracles to happen even if you have pregnancy complications.

It's not magic. It's not a theory. It's simply biology and how our bodies are built to work.

The relaxation response has been empirically tested so many times with consistent, reliable results of symptom improvement or even spontaneous remission of diseases that Dr. Benson considers it as predictably effective as taking a pill.[21] The relaxation response is something that you can activate at any time and can work up to 90% of the time when you know how to elicit it properly, and the effects are predictable every single time.[22]

Unlike a pill, it's naturally built inside of you, like an internal pharmacy, so you don't have to go anywhere to get it. It has no contraindications for any other medications or treatments you're taking. You can access it anytime you want, for free.

Allowing your body to activate its built-in self-repair system has profound implications for your health. Many research studies have shown that effectively relieving physical and emotional stress can help you stay pregnant longer, even if you are already experiencing pregnancy complications or are in preterm labor,[23] because of the balance that's restored among the endocrine, immune, and nervous systems.[24] In other words, activating the relaxation response does to your body during pregnancy what fixing the tilted domino does to the pattern you've created. It works as it's supposed to.

Learning this all of this and how it impacts pregnancy left me speechless, breathless, and completely dizzy. If we have such a powerful system in our bodies that is designed to help us heal and help us stay pregnant, why is this not being shouted from the rooftops? Why is this not part of every health class, every fertility clinic's initial consultation, every appointment with your OB or high-risk OB?

The truth: It doesn't cost anything, so pharmaceutical companies do not want this information to be public knowledge. In addition, there is still tremendous resistance among the medical field about this connection, despite years of evidence proving otherwise, and there are three major reasons why.

Hundreds of years ago, French philosopher René Descartes announced that the mind and body do exist and function independently, saying that because we cannot see or touch the mind, it cannot be connected to a physical body.[25] His pronouncements became the foundation of what we know today as Western medicine. This is deeply ingrained in traditional medical training as well as how we raise our children. From a young age, we are taught that mind and body are separate. We search for physical causes for our physical symptoms, only rarely considering they may have a mental component or root to them. Even insurance companies have different levels of coverage for medical and mental health.

Mind-body and psychoneuroimmunology research is also slow to be adapted into standard medical practice for another reason. While there is tremendous literature already in existence, far more data needs to be collected. However, not all associations, correlations, and connections in health can be empirically proven, because to gather such evidence would require conducting research studies that are unethical. There are plenty of empirical studies that would be extremely beneficial to lead to learn more about the cause of conditions such as preterm premature rupture of membranes (PPROM), incompetent cervix, or preterm labor—but they would never be approved by the institutional review board of any research institution today because of the harm it could do to women and their babies during pregnancy to conduct a research study of that kind. Because of this, many medical professionals then incorrectly interpret the lack of data as a nonexistent connection between stress and pregnancy complications.

This, then, leads to the third reason why there is so much resistance to accepting the power of the mind-body connection, especially in pregnancy: It's often lumped under the category of "alternative medicine," which includes interventions such as acupuncture, acupressure, and herbal remedies. In lay terms, as well as among the medical community, alternative medicine refers to anything other than Western medication, medical interventions, or surgery. The reaction to alternative medicine is often a hand-waving from many Western medicine practitioners who question its true impact on improving pregnancy health, citing it as not "evidence-based."

As journalist Jo Marchant put it so perfectly, "Terms like 'mind-body' and 'holistic' are often derided as flaky and unscientific, but in fact it's the idea of a mind distinct from the body, an ephemeral entity that floats somewhere in the skull like a spirit or a soul, that makes no scientific sense."[26]

What many medical professionals are unaware of is that the mind-body literature *is* evidence-based, with studies conducted as rigorously as any others within Western medicine.[27] The bigger issue is that the results of these studies deeply and profoundly challenge what we know to be true about health, wellness, and prenatal care, and that's hard for a lot of people to accept, professionals and patients alike.

When you accept that your body is created with a natural repair system that's designed to help you achieve and maintain health, and achieve and sustain pregnancy, suddenly the way you view your body and what's possible for your health and the health of your baby completely changes.

Let's be careful, however, in assuming that mind-body medicine and traditional Western medicine are mutually exclusive. Yes, we have a self-healing mechanism built into our bodies, but not all health conditions can be healed simply by our bodies alone. We do still need access to medical advancements such as surgeries, antibiotics, and tocolytics (medications to stop preterm contractions). However, these interventions and treatments also are more effective when your self-healing system is activated. Mind-body and Western medicine aren't at odds. They are both essential and need each other to be most effective at helping you be at your healthiest during your high-risk pregnancy.

As I continued my research into the depths of stress, pregnancy, and the mind-body connection, I kept thinking about all the women who are struggling in silence, feeling helpless to do anything to protect their baby during a high-risk pregnancy but wishing they could do something—*anything*—to give their baby a strong start to life. Women who have been kept in the dark about this profound and powerful mind-body connection.

I know, because I was one of those women. I had a very difficult pregnancy and became one of those miracle stories you hear about. There's nothing in the medical literature that explains why I stayed pregnant with all of the complications I faced. There's nothing inherently special about me or my pregnancy that explains it either. None of it makes sense until you look at the mind-body work of so many pioneers who have staked their lives and careers on the line to say this: There is a deep mind-body connection that impacts the health of your pregnancy, how long you stay pregnant, and ultimately the health of your baby.

If this sounds like a bunch of magic and fluffy, woo-woo claims, I understand. So few doctors discuss this with their patients that it's hard to believe the handful of scientists and practitioners who are speaking out could be right. But the proof is there. The data is there. The science is there. And the real-life miracle stories are there too.[28]

You're reading this book because you're likely going through a high-risk pregnancy yourself. That means one or more of the following apply to you:

- You are over the age of 35.
- You have pregnancy complications currently.
- You have a history of pregnancies with complications
- You are pregnant after fertility treatment.
- You have a history of preterm delivery.
- You have a history of medical problems (like asthma, autoimmune disease, kidney disease, cancer, etc.).
- You have a history of recurrent pregnancy loss.
- You have delivered a stillborn child (or children) in the past.

If you're reading this and going through a high-risk pregnancy, you're probably also overwhelmed with data, statistics, diagnoses, and prognoses that are making the hamster wheel in your head spin out of control. That's why, instead of this book being a clinical guide on the mind-body science of a healthy pregnancy, I wrote this book as a conversation, as if you and I are sitting at your kitchen table, having tea, and talking about how to help you through this difficult time.

Throughout this book, we will discuss how you can activate the relaxation response that's built into your body. I'll show you how this is possible whether you're on hospital bed rest in the middle of a medical crisis or at at work feeling worried about a test result or lying awake in the middle of the night because you can't fall back asleep after getting up to use the bathroom for the 75th time.

I'll share with you my story of my very high-risk pregnancy as well as the stories of many women I have helped who experienced their own miracles by relying on the powerful mind-body connection to show you how it works in real life outside of theory and the laboratory. I use my journey as a vessel through which to show you just how much the stress and relaxation responses impact your pregnancy, for better or for worse. I bring you into my world during some of the hardest months of my life to show you that you have more power than you realize during your pregnancy. I invite you into that chapter of my family-building journey to help you see how you can create your own miracles, too. I'm not a believer because my story has a happy ending. I'm a believer because data, tools, and research exist to help women have healthier pregnancies—and they cannot be hidden from women any longer. In the appendices, I share with you some of my favorite tools and strategies you can try yourself to help you experience for yourself the power of your mind and your body during a high-risk pregnancy.

If you're like me and skeptical of outrageous claims that sound like magic, I also share with you scientific evidence for why the mind-body connection works, why it worked for me, and why it can work for you too. In the back of the book, you'll find a list research and resources to do your own digging and discover the scientific proof that you can help yourself have a healthy high-risk pregnancy, even if you have pregnancy complications.

Two more things before we jump in:

First, nothing I share here is meant to advise about any particular medical treatment. That is decided between you and your treating physician. Just because one particular medical intervention worked for me, doesn't mean it will work for you, or vice versa. I only share the specifics of my particular journey to show you how you can use the mind-body connection to help you during *your* specific pregnancy.

Second, what I share with you might trigger a lot of deep, intense feelings. My journey to bringing my son home challenges a lot of commonly held beliefs about medicine, prenatal care, and what's in our control during pregnancy. It might bring up feelings of guilt about past losses. It might raise doubts about whether you were at fault for what you've been through before or are going through right now. It might bring up feelings of anger or resentment toward me for sharing this. You might want to put the book away because you think miracles can't happen for you too. You might even think I'm making some of this up, conveniently making it fit for my story and my journey.

Whatever you feel, allow yourself to feel it.

But most importantly, know that I don't blame you for anything you've been through. You are not at fault for your losses, your difficulty getting pregnant, your pregnancy complications, your preterm deliveries, or your babies with medical complications.

None of it is your fault. I invite you to believe that with every fiber of your being, too.

I wrote this book for you, the strong, intelligent woman who is determined to fight for her baby's life. I wrote it for you, the powerhouse woman who's been made to feel helpless during your pregnancy when your inner mama bear wants to do everything in your power to protect your little one. I wrote it for you because I know that there is so much that is in your control to manage your complications and have a healthier pregnancy so you can give your baby a strong start to life.

My sincere hope is that you, after reading this book, realize miracles don't just happen "out there" to "other people." I hope by the end of this book you can feel in your bones that you can stack the odds in your favor so that miracles can happen for you, too.

As you read this book, I just ask that you keep an open mind. Allow yourself to be blown away by the power that lies in your body. Give yourself permission to see outside the traditional box of possibilities during a high-risk pregnancy, and release the old beliefs that there's nothing you can do to help yourself and your baby during pregnancy. Be bold and take back control of your health.

I believe miracles can happen for you, too. I really do, with all my heart. I can't wait for you to join me.

CHAPTER 1

Miracles Start in the Mind

Miracles are not contrary to nature,
but only contrary to what we know about nature.

—AUGUSTINE OF HIPPO

"It's going to be a miracle if we can have kids," I grumbled to Sonil, my husband, one evening as I was giving myself an injection for our in vitro fertilization (IVF) cycle. I said that word, *miracle,* as if it was something I was allergic to. Something that happened to other people, not me. Like winning the lottery.

The heaviness of that reality hadn't really sunk in, but the words were pouring out. My mouth, though, had filtered out some of the darker thoughts that were floating in my head.

What if not being able to get pregnant was a sign that I shouldn't be a mother? What if I would be a horrible mother? Maybe I'd mess up my children and this is Mother Nature's way of preventing that from happening.

Hi, I'm Parijat.

Being dramatic is one of my superpowers.

Another superpower? Being a perfectionist.

Since I was young, I have strived for perfection. When I work hard, I get results. When I put in the right type of work, I get the best results. Nothing but the best was good enough, and if I got anything less than the best, I went back to my books and studied harder, longer, focused more, to do my best.

I'm the kid who scolded myself for getting a 97% on a test when my parents were thrilled for me.

I'm the kid who created quizzes for myself every Friday afternoon to see if I had yet mastered being able to write out the Marathi alphabet so that when I went to India a few weeks later, I'd be able to read the signs.

I was a Type A+.

While this strong work ethic led to tremendous academic and career success very early in my life, I learned the hard way that fertility and pregnancy didn't work like that.

I was healthy. I exercised. I ate well. I was happy. I got plenty of sleep at night. But after our first round of fertility treatment, I lost the baby due to a ruptured ectopic.

Internal bleeding. My doctor reassuring us that I would survive. Emergency surgery to remove my ruptured fallopian tube and the first baby I carried.

I felt broken and I doubted whether I could carry another pregnancy. I felt insecure in my body. The grief and guilt of losing a baby that had been there and was growing, until it outgrew its home, sat deep in my bones.

I recovered physically in a couple of months and emotionally several months after that. We were ready to try again, hoping this baby would stick and be the baby we got to bring home, but the dark clouds loomed over us.

We were told grim statistics. In vitro fertilization was not a sure shot. It wasn't the 100% chance of success we expected. Not for us. Not for anyone. We knew we could experience another ectopic pregnancy. I could experience a miscarriage. It could just be a failed cycle with a negative pregnancy test.

Still, we decided to go forward and hope the statistics were in our favor. I entered hormone bootcamp, and Sonil learned what it was like to live with a monster at home while also learning how to become an apothecary.

I don't know which he hated more.

"This is idiot-proof," I'd tell him every night as looked on with worry.

He'd kneel by the nightstand, the bedside lamp glowing over the syringes and tubes as he mixed the tincture of powder with saline and filled up a syringe with fertility medications. "If there wasn't a *gigantic* margin of error they'd never let us do this ourselves."

He'd laugh wryly—just to make me feel better—but still look at the syringe 15 more times under the warm yellow hue of the lamp, making sure it was filled *exactly* to 1mL before handing it to me to inject in my stomach.

He'd cringe as I injected myself, shouting cheers while I held my breath as the medicine burned when going in.

"You can do it! You've got this, P!" he'd say every single night, to which I'd roll my eyes and ask if he was ready to grow some ovaries for us yet because I was never going to do this again.

The next night, we'd repeat the ritual the exact same way.

On a hot morning in May, we were ready for our very first embryo transfer. Having hope again and staying positive were two challenges we faced. We had both been traumatized by the ruptured ectopic and were fiercely guarding our hearts for more devastation as we moved forward.

The drive to the fertility clinic that morning was smooth. I looked out the window and noticed the beautiful green hills looking strong and majestic. They brought a sense of peace. I thought maybe that could be a sign for how easy the rest of this process was going to be and, before we knew it, we'd have a baby to bring home. I took any signs I could get.

We pulled into the parking lot of the clinic and, as we walked into the waiting room, we instinctively held our breaths.

"I can't look. You look," I whispered to Sonil as we entered the waiting area.

I heard him audibly breathe out and whisper back, "It's off."

"Oh thank goodness!" I sighed out of relief and opened my eyes to see that the TV was indeed off.

Every single time we had come prior to this day, the movie *Secretariat* had been playing. For every appointment, every ultrasound, every meeting, we'd walk in and see that horse galloping away on the screen with no care in the world. Every single one of those appointments had resulted in bad news. It obviously wasn't the fault of the movie, but I had developed a deep resentment toward that horse.

It was a relief to see that movie wasn't on that day. Maybe another sign that things would go smoothly for us from here on out?

Both Sonil and I come from strong research backgrounds—though totally different fields—with a value for data, statistics, facts, and numbers. We were both very clinical and logical about our views of the world, for better or for worse. But infertility had begun to challenge that and was molding us into vastly different people than we had been prior to fertility treatment, one habit at a time.

Specifically, we'd become superstitious about where to sit in the waiting room. We scanned the room and saw a variety of couples sitting together. Some women were leaning on their partners, looking like they were in discomfort. Some couples were whispering very quietly under their breath, hoping not to draw attention. Others were playing separately on their phones waiting for their names to be called.

There were two seats together in the corner. We looked at each other and shook our heads fervently. No way were we sitting there. That's where we sat when we found out my fallopian tube had ruptured and I needed emergency surgery. Those chairs carry bad memories— and bad luck.

Sonil started walking toward the middle of the room and I followed, not knowing the plan he had in mind. As he was about to sit, he pointed to another chair for me—on the exact opposite side of the waiting area.

It was a great plan. We'd never sat like that before.

We also looked like idiots.

More accurately, we looked like a couple who couldn't stand each other. Who were we to try to have a baby when we couldn't even sit next to each other? It looked like we needed a referral to couples counseling instead of an appointment with a fertility doctor! I had to hide my face behind a magazine to keep from laughing at the absurdity of it all.

That's just how we dealt, one superstitious decision at a time, and I knew we weren't alone.

ᴗ

We've all done it throughout our lives at some point: the lucky jersey for the biggest game of the season. The special pencil for the hardest test of the semester. Parking in a certain part of the garage before a big presentation. Rabbits' feet. Four-leaf clovers. Blowing on dandelions. We all look for our lucky charms and create some superstitious ritual around us. It's human to try to make sense from what seems like chaos.

Many couples feel helpless when there is so much that is unknown about fertility and pregnancy. You start to make up a story to create a sense of cause and effect. Superstition becomes the norm. It's the only way to establish a sense of predictability and sanity—some sense of control. It's the only way we know how to hope for a miracle.

Medical miracles are a whole other beast, though. If winning the lottery feels hard, beating the odds for a health condition can seem downright impossible because we assign the word *miracle* to something people can't explain. You've heard stories of medical miracles. Like the story of a woman whose stage-four cancer went into remission even when she was given one month to live. Or the man whose kidneys started spontaneously working when he had been on dialysis for weeks. Or the woman whose chronic illness reversed and disappeared almost magically. Or the woman who delivered at term despite dozens of complications and threatened preterm delivery. Or the 22-weeker who weighed less than 1 pound who is a thriving toddler.

We all hear stories like this and think, *Wow. What a stroke of luck.* Or *God was watching down on her.* Or *His angels pulled him through.*

Or sometimes we just shrug our shoulders and say that there was no rhyme or reason (but then encourage her to buy a lotto ticket).

It seems like medical miracles are as random as the slot machines in Las Vegas. But when you look a little closer at how our bodies work, these medical miracles start to make more sense, making you think, and then *believe*, that maybe they can happen to you too.

In fact, that's the key right there. That one word. *Belief.*

To experience a medical miracle requires you to answer one question with a strong, resounding yes: *Do you believe you can experience a miracle during this pregnancy?* That can mean anything to you: making it through the first trimester, staying pregnant longer than any of your previous pregnancies, bringing the baby home. A miracle is whatever you consider it to be. The question is: *Do you believe it's possible for it to happen to you?*

The answer can't be a fake-it-'til-you-make-it *yes*. You can't try to convince yourself to believe it to be true. This is not a blind belief that you hope turns into reality. It needs to be a solid, I-believe-this-with-all-my-heart *HELL YES!*

Miracles begin in the mind. Miracles happen because you believe they're possible. Miracles happen because you believe your body can do something even science says you cannot. That strong belief comes when you fully embrace that we are infinitely powerful in impacting our health, even during a high-risk pregnancy.

I know it sounds fluffy and New Age-y. You're probably half-expecting me to start talking about planets aligning with the stars and crystals hanging above your bed. (No judgment if you believe in that!) But that's not what this is. This is plain and simple biology. When you believe (not think, but really, truly believe) that positive outcomes can happen for you, physiological changes happen in your body.

I'll be honest: Having an unwavering belief that your mind can have a profound impact on your pregnancy, especially when you're high-risk, is hard. It goes against a lot of what you're likely hearing from your doctor about what's possible during your pregnancy. It also probably goes against how you're feeling about your body during your pregnancy—feeling broken and wondering why being pregnant is so much more challenging for you than it is for other women.

Not believing with every fiber of your being that miracles can happen for you leaves you feeling like you're at the mercy of a body that's gone rogue. You feel out of control, constantly waiting for the other shoe to drop. You start imagining worst-case scenarios, your mind going adrift like a boat in the ocean without an anchor. That feeling of helplessness activates the stress response in your body.

Having a healthy high-risk pregnancy requires turning off the stress response as often as possible so your self-healing system can help you heal. To do this starts with making a conscious choice to believe that your body is capable of keeping your baby safe, that *you* are capable of keeping your baby safe. Turning off the stress response and turning on the relaxation response involves changing the script about your body and what it's doing.

It's easy to believe that your body is doing whatever it wants, is failing you, or is broken. You'll see throughout the book how often and how deeply I believed that, especially during our most challenging moments. During pregnancy, however, our body is naturally built to keep us and our babies safe for as long as possible. To be able to do that, requires a staunch determination to create a physical environment in which your body can do what it does best. The key to that is the relaxation response, and the first step to activating it is to believe you have a built-in repair system and that activating it can actually help you have a healthy pregnancy.

This is different than thinking "everything will be okay." In fact, positive thinking is not nearly as helpful as we like to believe because thoughts are fleeting. Thoughts are created by you in response to your mood, your habits, and your current physical state. (Ever have positive thoughts when you're hangry?)

As I tell my clients, you can talk yourself in and out of anything and those thoughts feel like facts when they're not. But believing something to be true, that's a different ballgame. This belief often has no words. It's a gut feeling or something you feel in your bones. It's something you know to be true without needing evidence or hard facts.

So again I ask: *Do you believe the built-in repair system in your body can help you and your baby experience a miracle during this pregnancy?*

At this point, you might be wondering if this is all real or just a placebo effect.[1] Is the relaxation response just something that's "in your head" and it just "happens" to work? These were my questions as well when I first learned about it, so let's set the record straight.

The placebo effect *is* when you believe something will help you and then it does. For example, your doctor gives you a pill and says it's a pain medication that will cure you of your headache. You take it, not realizing it's just a sugar pill, and your headache goes away. That is the placebo effect. So yes, in a way, it is in your head.

That's not *just* it, though. The placebo effect is not about wishing or willing your pregnancy complications away. It's about believing that whatever you're doing to try to manage them will help. In this example, believing that pill will help you is not about the pill as much as it is about the belief about the effectiveness of the pill. With regard to your pregnancy, it's about believing that your body has a built-in repair system that can help you stay pregnant and have a healthy baby.

This belief creates physiological changes down to the cellular level that we call the placebo effect. The result (your headache disappearing or your complications improving) is not just "in your head" but a psychological effect that cascades into your body.[2] By changing hormonal, neural, and immunological pathways that are essential for helping you activate the relaxation response and turn off the stress response, your body is able to focus on helping you stay pregnant. As Dr. Bruce Lipton says, "Belief changes biology!"[3]

What does all of this mean in plain English?

Medical miracles start in your head. Whether something will work for you during your high-risk pregnancy to help you stay pregnant—whether it's medicine, surgeries, or the built-in repair system in your body—starts with you believing it will work. Your body can change because you *believe* it can change. Your blood pressure can come down if you *believe* it can come down. Your blood glucose levels can stabilize because you *believe* they can stabilize. Your preterm contractions can slow or stop because you *believe* they can slow or stop.

Belief alone isn't enough to manage your complications, of course, but it is the critical first step.

*

The embryology report for that day was great. Ten embryos had survived to that day.

Sonil and I raised our eyebrows at each other. We weren't even parents yet technically, but we were still proud of the little brood we had created!

My reproductive endocrinologist (RE), whom I'll call Dr. Davidson, continued that, of the 10, three of them looked really strong.

"Here's the one we're transfering today," he said as he handed me a picture of a day three embryo. *Our* embryo! It looked just perfect.

The catheter with the embryo in it was threaded through my cervix, and on a black flat-screen TV mounted on the side of the room, we saw this little white shining star shoot into my uterus.

"There it is!" Dr. Davidson said, as if this was his first transfer too.

The magic of this moment wasn't lost on even the professionals who do this day in and day out.

I grabbed and squeezed Sonil's hand so tight. Our sarcastic humor and our tamed expectations had gone out the window. Hope was overflowing. Unforced. Unfiltered. Totally genuine.

We had no idea if this embryo would implant (transferring an embryo into the uterus does not guarantee implantation into the uterine lining), but we had so much hope for our future.

Please hang on. Please get comfortable, I thought. *Please make this your home for the next nine months. I can't wait to meet you early next year.*

The ride home was peaceful as we embraced hope. All the data, statistics, numbers that we'd gone over at length with Dr. Davidson just a few days prior were nowhere to be found in our minds.

Who were these giddy, hopeful, optimistic people who usually made sarcastic jokes and thrived on dark humor?

❧

Hope is an interesting emotion. It's often said that it's the emotion that keeps us alive. It doesn't knock, waiting to be let in. It enters on its own. It makes itself at home, and you have to work really, really hard to kick it out. Our bodies are naturally inclined to have hope, because physiologically it creates and maintains the changes in your body that you need for your body to function optimally. Simply put, hope is not just a positive mental state. Feeling hope creates biochemical changes in the body that deeply impact your immune system, hormones, and your nervous system.[4] That domino game we talked about earlier? Hope keeps the pieces in line so the game can continue the way it should.

If you do kick hope out, though (which I have done many times, as you'll see), it's replaced by fear, stress, and anxiety—everything that stops your body from working optimally because the focus becomes about self-preservation and survival.

Hope is one of the strongest facilitators of the relaxation system that's necessary to help you get pregnant[5] and stay pregnant even if you have complications. (We'll review this in more detail in Chapter 8.)

❦

On the drive home, we allowed ourselves to surrender to hope, believing that this could be our miracle and our baby we get to bring home.

"We need to give the embryo a name," I blurted out, turning down the volume of the horrible pop music we were listening to on the radio.

Sonil was completely confused.

I had read about this tradition on some infertility blogs and had become obsessed with it over the previous few months. Couples would give their embryos a nickname at the time of transfer. I loved how it helped couples bond with a little pack of cells as they waited to find out if the embryo implanted or not.

He was on a hope high so he readily agreed.

True to his style, he started throwing out some crazy ideas:

Ninja.
Cloud 9.
Peanut butter.

"Peanut butter?!?" I yelled. "I'm allergic to peanut butter! Is that the kind of message you want to send to this baby and my body already?!"

We laughed at the absurdity of all of this but kept playing anyway.

Truth be told, the lightness of this moment was a much-needed experience.

We were getting reacquainted to light after months of darkness and grief. I was getting used to my body feeling relaxed and comfortable.

We went back and forth with some ideas, and finally I asked, "How about MB?"

"What the heck does that mean?"

I explained to him that in the infertility world, an embryo is often nicknamed an "embie."

"Richard, Richie. Embryo, Embie. Get it?"

"Ohhh, okay."

"So what if we played off of that but did the letters M and B? MB?"

Being a huge fan of puns and play on words, Sonil immediately loved it. For at least the next two weeks, while we waited to take a pregnancy test (and, we hoped, for many months after), this little embryo was to be called MB.

We had no idea how meaningful that name would become and how much it would give us the hope we needed to fight for this little life.

*

According to professor Norman Cousins, "[T]he mind of the patient creates the ambience of treatment. Belief becomes biology. The head comes first."[6]

So before you continue any further, take a moment and answer these questions:

- Where is your head? What types of thoughts are you thinking to yourself?
- Are you hopeful that this is the baby you'll get to bring home?
- Do you believe your body can do its very best to keep you and your baby safe?
- Is your head in the right space to give your body (and the medical treatment you're receiving) the very best chance at creating miracles? If it's not, what do you need to get it there? What's holding you back?

- What benefit is it serving you to hold onto the story you're telling yourself about your body, your pregnancy, and what's possible for you?

Journaling through these questions can help clarify where your thoughts are getting stuck and what you need to do to believe, wholeheartedly, that miracles can happen for you too.

Remember: Before any tool you can learn to relieve stress, your belief that you can protect this baby during this pregnancy has to come first.

CHAPTER 2

Building the Right Village

The process of finding the right doctor for you is excruciatingly painful, sometimes causing more damage than what you started with, but the feeling of finding the right one is priceless.

—PRUDENCE HAYES

How much do you trust your OB?

I ask this question to almost all of my clients and it often takes them by surprise. Why would I ask a question that has such an obvious answer?

"I trust him/her with my life" is frequently what I hear. Not always, but often.

My intention with asking the question is not to find out how much they trust their doctor's medical expertise, but how much they trust their doctor to *care* about them as human beings with complex feelings and who are trying to cope with the uncertainties of a high-risk pregnancy. I also want to know how much they trust their doctors to have a positive outlook on their prognosis even if the data proves otherwise. When I phrase the question again like that, many of them change their answers.

While most of the women I speak with trust their doctor's

medical advice, few of them feel like their OB understands or is interested in their personal experience of living with a high-risk pregnancy. They feel like their OB does not know how to provide the support that's required to cope with the uncertainties.

This doesn't surprise me. Take a moment to think about this. . . .

How often does your doctor check your blood pressure, your fundal height, your cervical length? And how often does she/he ask you how you're feeling or coping with your high-risk pregnancy? For most women, the answers are: every appointment and never, respectively.

Part of the reason is because physicians don't have time to get into it. With the current state of our medical system, doctors spend an average of 13–16 minutes with each patient,[1] leaving patients feeling like nothing more than a case number or an item on a to-do list. Far too many women tell me that they feel rushed in their appointments and don't have enough time to ask all of their questions. What's worse, they feel their concerns are often waved off as "just anxiety."

Another reason doctors fail to ask about how you're coping with a high-risk pregnancy is because they don't have the training on how to support a woman emotionally through a health crisis like a high-risk pregnancy. They may be kind, loving, warm people, but medical training also splits the education between the mind and body at a very early stage, leaving them without the tools and skills to adequately help even if they were to inquire about your mental or emotional state. "Everything's fine," women tell me their doctor reassures them, as if those two words will immediately diminish their anxiety. In other cases, doctors offer medication, which many women I speak with don't wish to take during pregnancy for a variety of reasons, to ease the anxiety. The end result is the same: Women end up feeling helpless and like they just have to ride the wave of anxiety and fear until the baby comes home.

That does not have to be your experience during your pregnancy. It starts with ensuring you have the right professionals on your prenatal team to care for you and baby through your pregnancy. This is important because your relationship with your doctor plays a tremendous role in your stress levels during your high-risk pregnancy. It's not the words your OB uses that turns on your stress response as much as how your doctor shows up in the room, spends time with you, answers your questions and shows you with their actions that they care. It's through the hope they convey for your future and your prognosis as well as the reassurance they provide you when you share your worries.

Research shows having a strong prenatal team is not just about having doctors and nurses who are highly educated or specially trained to treat your medical complication(s). A strong prenatal team involves medical professionals who help you feel cared for and who encourage hope despite low odds. Having this type of doctor on your medical team has a profound impact on your physical health.

Yes, you read that right. How your doctor treats you, how nurtured and cared for you feel by your medical team, as well as how they disclose bad news to you, actually impact your physical health.

Dr. Andrew Weil coined the term *medical hexing*,[2] which describes the phenomenon most women during a high-risk pregnancy experience. This is when a doctor shares bad news from a perspective that dashes hope for a positive prognosis. For example, he might tell you that your chances of making it to 32 weeks are slim. Or she might share statistics about why you're likely to develop a preeclampsia again this time around. It's not the bad news that's the issue; it's the delivery of the bad news, making you feel like it is your fate and there's no hope for any other outcome.

Conversations like these (that qualify as medical hexing) create a cascade of negative changes in the body by way of triggering the stress response. I have worked with too many clients who have shared that their doctor's "doom and gloom" attitude makes them feel more anxious after their appointments instead of feeling better. They notice these conversations negatively impact symptoms such as preterm contractions, blood pressure, and sleep, among others.

Finding a doctor who has good bedside manner is so much more than feeling comfortable in their presence. It's about finding someone who can walk the fine line of being honest, open, and realistic about your situation while also inspiring hope, faith, and belief that miracles can happen for you still. This right here highlights the art of medicine, something many doctors have mastered and many have not.

🌿

I was on the floor of my bathroom. I could feel the cold tile against my legs. My head leaned against the wall. I was breathing so fast I was feeling lightheaded. I had the phone pressed tightly against my ear.

"I'm bleeding. It's a lot," I told Dr. Davidson between sobs.

I described to him the huge clots that I had just passed and the sea of red that I had seen in the toilet.

I asked him—begged him—to tell me what was happening. I knew this wasn't normal. I was hardly six weeks along in my pregnancy. There was nothing normal about this.

Am I in the middle of a miscarriage? I know I didn't pass the tissue already. What's happening?

It felt like somebody was suffocating me as the tears fell down my face.

I was desperate. It was so early in the pregnancy and yet I had such a strong maternal instinct to protect this little life. I wasn't ready to lose it and I didn't know what was happening, but I wanted to do whatever I could to protect this little baby.

I waited for Dr. Davidson to answer. His voice was soft and quiet. I could feel his years of experience in the way that he spoke kindly with me. I could feel his heart in his work. He always made me feel like I was his only patient and that he personally cared about what happened for us.

I knew he could hear the desperation in my voice. I wasn't exactly doing anything to hide it. It's a desperation I'm sure he had heard in the voices of hundreds of women before who felt helpless while their bodies were doing things that didn't make any sense.

He offered to schedule an ultrasound the next day for peace of mind.

"If it's a miscarriage, there isn't anything we can do about it but you can come in and we can try to see if we can find out what's going on," he said gently.

Technically, just six weeks into the pregnancy was too soon for an ultrasound. Often, it's too early to even see a heartbeat. Because there are such a high number of false negatives that early in a pregnancy, most doctors don't call you in that soon. I appreciated the offer and I knew it would help me feel better to visualize what was happening on screen. I scheduled the appointment anyway, knowing we could be setting ourselves up for no news because it was too early.

The dark, hopeless thoughts from the pre-IVF days seeped back in.

I was sure we wouldn't see a heartbeat. I was convinced it was a miscarriage. I called Sonil and asked him to come home. I couldn't be by myself, especially if I was about to lose the baby.

I dragged myself off the bathroom floor, washed my hands, and made my way to the sofa. I turned on some mindless TV to try to drown out the voices in my head that were going through all of the horrible scenarios that could play out the next day.

Making lists upon lists of things that could go wrong. Imagining the worst-case scenario. My body was tense. I was hardly breathing. Hope was nowhere to be found.

Lizard brain. Grizzly bear. Run.

I closed my eyes and leaned my head against the sofa and tried to hear Dr. Davidson's voice in my head. He was confident we could figure out what was going on. Even if it was a miscarriage, I knew I was in good hands because I knew he was personally invested in us being able to have a baby. Whatever we would find, I knew he would talk me through it, as he always had through all of the ups and downs of my fertility journey thus far. He wouldn't hide any information from me. He would ask for my opinion, and trust it, on whatever health decisions needed to be made.

I was alone at home, but focusing on this was a much-needed reminder that I wasn't alone on this journey to fight for my baby.

Deep breaths. *We're in this together.*

I had come across Dr. Davidson's profile on his clinic's website several times before I got the courage to call him. No matter how many times I searched—by location, by clinic, by patient reviews—his name kept popping up, and I kept clicking away to continue my search. He looked intimidating. It wasn't so much because of his picture but moreso because of his multiple advanced degrees. They made me worry he'd have a huge ego and wouldn't listen to me when I shared my concerns. Too many experiences with doctors like that had left me jaded and untrusting of new specialists, especially when I knew my body did not have typical reactions to the most common medications.

In fact, I had just fired the doctor who had done my surgery to diagnose endometriosis for this very reason. At my final appointment with the surgeon, when I complained to him that my pain had become worse after starting the new treatment protocol, he said, "Well, endometriosis hurts," with a shrug of his shoulders.

I stared at him in disbelief.

That was his answer? He was going to just shrug his shoulders and leave the room without wanting to help or find another solution to reduce my pain? I was shocked. That one comment made me walk out the door of his office and never return.

That type of thinking and patient care was not at all in line with what I wanted from members of my medical team, especially when I knew getting pregnant was going to be a difficult and emotional journey. I wanted a doctor who was going to partner with me to solve my problems no matter how unsolvable research and data told him they were. I wanted a doctor who was going to trust me and keep fighting for me until we found a solution that returned some quality of life to me. I wanted a doctor who believed anything was possible if we trusted my body.

I did not want one who was going to shrug his shoulders and walk away leaving me to fend for myself. Nope. Not interested.

I was on the clock to find someone to replace him and manage my treatment because my pain and treatment side effects were getting worse. After several days of searching and calling clinics, being put on six-month waiting lists, and having my voice mails disappear into the void, I finally got the guts and called Dr. Davidson's office to make an appointment.

I was terrified to meet him.

Was he going to think I was crazy for seeing a fertility specialist in my 20s? Was he going to think I was over-exaggerating the problems I had? Was he going to brush me aside as an anxious person who relies on Google too much? I worried and prepared myself for a disappointing appointment.

Sonil and I met Dr. Davidson in his office, where he'd set up a computer with a PowerPoint presentation. That earned him one point right off the bat. (PowerPoint presentations speak to my nerd heart.)

After brief introductions, he went through the presentation, showing us how reproductive systems work, where mine was faulty (my word, not his), and why he recommended the treatment that he did to help preserve my fertility.

I was shocked at how meticulously he was explaining everything, as if his most important priority was us being educated about our bodies. He didn't talk down to us; he talked *with* us until we were on the same page and understood what was going on.

Two points, doctor.

I took pages of notes during that appointment and learned so much about my body that no one had ever spent time telling me about.

The nail in the coffin was what happened next. After he was done talking, I explained to him why I disagreed with his treatment recommendation. I had already tried it and had a very rare and unusual reaction to the medication.

I held my breath.

pregnancy brain.

He's going to be offended that I disagree. He's going to try to convince me I'm wrong and he's right. Here we go with the God complex.
I braced myself for it . . . but it didn't happen.
Instead, he asked questions: What were my side effects? When did they begin? What patterns did I notice that triggered the symptoms?
He admitted he hadn't heard about that type of reaction before, nor was it well-documented in the literature. Then, he thought for a moment and suggested a new treatment protocol that he thought was worth a try. It was out of the box, but he felt hopeful that it could bring me the relief I so desperately needed.
Jaw. Floor.
He showed me in the short, 30-minute consultation that I was not going to brave the unknown of infertility alone. I was sold.
Welcome to Team Parijat, Dr. Davidson. It's going to be a wild ride.

ᵍ

The doctor-patient relationship is a critical piece in the puzzle that explains spontaneous recovery, remission, and medical miracles. When you trust your doctor to have your back, to look for options that are beyond the obvious, to treat you as an individual patient and not just straight out of the book, and to tell you the difficult truth in the most compassionate, hopeful, and empowering way, it creates physiological changes in your body.

"When we are receiving medical care, our mental state matters. Those who feel alone and afraid do not fare as well as those who feel supported, safe and in control," Jo Marchant found when she dug into the decades of research about why having a caring medical team during a health crisis is critical to positive health outcomes.[3]

When you have a doctor on your team who cares about you, and who provides warmth and reassurance, especially when things feel like they are falling apart, changes happen in your body—physical, biological changes. Seeing or speaking with a doctor whom you trust turns off the physical stress response and triggers the relaxation response, which readjusts your immune system, endocrine system, and nervous system in a way that promotes healing and repair.

Think about a moment when you had a sore throat or a headache. You go see your doctor, whom you trust, only to have the symptoms disappear as soon as you are in the exam room. The mind-body connection is at work. Your mind is calming you down, creating a cascade effect in your body of relaxation, relief, and repair. Pain improves, inflammation decreases, and you feel better. This is not a metaphysical change that occurs but actual shifts in your immune, neurological, and endocrine systems because of the relaxation response.

Does that mean your sore throat or headache was all in your head? No. You still have a cold that your doctor will diagnose. Is the activation of the relaxation response curing you of your headache or sore throat? Also no. It is setting up the physiological changes in your body that are necessary to help you fight off the infection or calm your nervous system to manage the pain. Our bodies have a built-in internal pharmacy that we tap into in order to do just that,[4] whether you have a cold or pregnancy complications.

On the flip side, ever go to see a doctor you don't feel totally comfortable around or you know you won't get a lot of time with to discuss your most pressing concerns? You might notice your pulse is higher than normal, your blood pressure is elevated, or you're breathing faster and sweating. The mind-body connection is at work here too. Your emotional and mental experience of your doctor is triggering the stress response. When you're in that physical and emotional state, your body cannot focus on repairing and healing the underlying cause of your symptoms, such as preterm contractions, elevated blood glucose levels, or high blood pressure.

What's worse is that when your stress response is on, whatever medications, supplements, or treatments your doctor suggests also work less effectively! The flip side is also true. When you work with a doctor whom you trust, who provides hope and thinks outside the box to help you with whatever complications lie ahead of you, the medical treatments they recommend will work more effectively. This happens because your relaxation response is on.

In a research study on the effectiveness of acupuncture for irritable bowel syndrome, 62% of participants experienced symptom relief when they received acupuncture treatment and their doctor developed a warm and attentive relationship, compared to 44% who received the same acupuncture treatment without a nurturing, personal relationship with their provider.[5] The only thing different between those groups was the relationship with the provider.

Additionally, when you feel stressed around your doctor, as opposed to supported or cared for, trust erodes. Research has shown that when patients don't trust their doctor, they experience significantly more side effects, even if all they're taking is vitamins.[6] Also, patients who don't trust their doctor are less likely to follow their physician's recommendations for treatment and care, not believing in the effectiveness. I can't tell you how often I have women divulge that they've put themselves on bed rest, even though their doctor told them it wasn't necessary, because they didn't believe their doctor understood the severity of the symptoms or concerns.

This highlights another mind-body effect that we fail to give credence to when it comes to health prognoses. It's what scientists call the *nocebo effect*. While the placebo effect demonstrates the power of hope, positive belief, and nurturing care on your health and prognosis, the nocebo effect demonstrates the power of negative belief on health outcomes.

The nocebo effect is so powerful that when cancer patients were given nothing but sugar water and were told that the "medication" would make them vomit, 80% of them did, even though none of them actually received medication.[7] This same effect occurs when you distrust your providers and/or the treatment they recommend. It also occurs when your doctor doesn't believe the treatment they recommend will help or when they believe nothing can be done to alleviate your symptoms or improve your condition.[8]

This nocebo effect has been shown to be particularly impactful and powerful for women who are pregnant. Researchers found that by the time women attended childbirth classes, they were already fearful and stressed about labor and delivery because of the months they had spent hearing scary stories from friends and family about what to expect. When asked, women typically expect an awful experience with labor and delivery and believe there's nothing they can do to change that. Midwives and doulas frequently report a stalling of labor, prolonged labor, and a higher incidence of c-sections when women experience stress and fear during delivery.[9]

Simply being labeled "high-risk" can trigger a nocebo effect, too, in some women who believe it's a sign of bad things to come for her and baby. This is especially true for women whose doctors have not reassured them otherwise.[10] Especially when you are high-risk, many appointments and conversations focus in what's going wrong in the pregnancy, which can also trigger the stress response through the nocebo effect.

You've probably heard stories about this from your friends, or experienced this yourself: Your doctor might quickly mention during an appointment that your baby is too big and you might need a c-section. You have gestational diabetes so you're likely to have a big baby. The baby's measuring a bit small, you should increase your caloric intake.

Most women, when they hear an off-handed comment like that, begin to feel anxious. Who wouldn't? You trust your doctor. You believe that they have your best interest at heart (and most of them do), but you can't help but worry about everything that could go wrong because of one comment in your appointment. You imagine losing choices with your birth plan and delivery experience. You begin to worry that something will be wrong with your baby, or your body, even if you ask your doctor and they reassure you that they're not worried—to just wait and see what happens and to not stress about it. Even if you can get yourself to think positively, guess what's happening in your body anyway: The stress response is on and your body is in self-protective mode.

Research shows that when a doctor plants the seed of negative expectations by suggesting (or clearly stating) that you likely won't stay pregnant until a certain milestone, or you're likely to lose the baby, or your might need a cesarean section to deliver your baby, it impacts your body profoundly. How a doctor presents a treatment and diagnosis impacts how *you* understand your health condition, treatment, and prognosis. If you received a diagnosis of a health complication or bad news from test results for you or your baby during your pregnancy and you feel like it's a sign of bad news for either of you or you have that "doom and gloom" feeling, it kicks off the stress response. It's your brain's way of telling your body you're in danger and the priority is to get to safety. Repair, recovery, and healing are no longer important or possible, increasing your risk of developing pregnancy complications and exacerbating symptoms for the complication you already have.

However, the solution to reduce that stress is not to pretend everything is fine or to think the statistics your doctor shared with you don't apply or are exaggerations of your reality. Despite the physical impact of the nocebo effect, ignorance is still not bliss.

The solution is for you *and* your physician to view that same diagnosis or test result as a challenge that you can overcome together. If you experience hope for a positive outcome despite the statistics your doctor is required to share with you, your body goes through an entirely different physiological experience. The relaxation response turns on. Your body's natural repair systems start to work, and that enhances the effectiveness of any treatment that your doctor recommends to help you manage your pregnancy complication.

Which experience you have depends largely on how your doctor presents the diagnosis or test results. Do you feel your doctor views this as a challenge that you can overcome together, even if the statistics are stacked against you? Or do you feel like your doctor has given up hope?

I worked with a client who was referred to me because she left every appointment with her OB in tears and with anxiety so high she couldn't sleep at night. She said that her doctor was sharing such scary statistics with her that she was convinced her baby was going to die. However, when I spoke with her OB (with my client's permission) he was shocked that was the message his patient was taking away from their conversations. He was merely sharing with her the statistics and likelihood of her miscarrying given her history. The data was real and it was absolutely applicable to her situation. But all she heard was "Your baby might die." It made perfect sense that her anxiety was through the roof. This anxiety presented as constant aches and pains, insomnia, trouble with digestion, and many more physical symptoms that she had never experienced before.

Our work together focused on helping her manage her anxiety effectively (which we'll discuss more in Chapter 3) as well as helping her experience how much she could influence her body and thus help her baby with small shifts she made daily. It renewed hope for her that this could be her take-home baby, elevated her mood, reduced her aches and pains, improved her sleep, and dissipated her anxiety. It also strengthened her relationship with her physician because she was able to lead the conversations from "doom and gloom" to viewing her situation as a challenge they could both work together to improve. Their conversations became productive about what she and her physician could do to alleviate her symptoms medically and increase her chances of staying pregnant and what she could do on her own at home to elevate those chances further. She finally started leaving the appointments with hope instead of dread and tears.

Another client was tremendously frustrated by her doctor's insistence to begin insulin without discussing lifestyle changes that could improve her blood glucose levels. She felt helpless and cornered and like she had no choices. After one session together with me, she developed the confidence to find a new high-risk OB. During that first appointment with him, he sat down with her for 30 minutes and answered all of her questions without rushing out of the room. After the appointment, her blood glucose levels were the lowest she had recorded since her diagnosis of gestational diabetes. Nothing in her treatment protocol had changed at that point.

One more reached out to me because she was starting to feel hopeless and depressed by the short visits she was having with her physician, who repeatedly told her to prepare for a preterm delivery without guarantee that her baby would survive. Yes, the statistics showed that delivering preterm was very likely given her particular complications. Depending on how prematurely she had the baby, there was a good chance he wouldn't have survived. Her doctor was being very realistic with her. But to her, the conversations felt cold and clinical, like her doctor had already given up hope. Without fail, after every appointment with him, she would experience a spike in contractions that lasted for hours at home. When we began working together, I taught her how to slow those contractions until she was able to find a new doctor to consult. This doctor shared the same statistics but in a productive way, such that she left every appointment with a plan, and never again did she experience preterm contractions after her appointments.

I could go on and on citing research and client stories that show this profound effect of the doctor-patient relationship on your health, but let's be honest: You don't need the research. You know all of this already. You know how much better you feel physically and emotionally when you're around a doctor who cares and provides attentive support, who believes anything is possible even when they are giving you bad news, and who trusts you and treats you as part of the team that, together, is going to overcome whatever challenge lies in front of you right now.

You also know how you feel when that doesn't happen. When you are waiting for days or weeks to see a physician, only for them to run in, barely make eye contact, listen while they're typing, and run out in a matter of minutes. You're left with unanswered questions and frustrated by the lack of care. You know how it feels when you hear your doctor's voice drop as they tell you there's nothing more that can be done, who talks as if they've given up hope and are preparing you to do the same.

It's in your hands to choose the right people to be on your medical team, to fight with you as you fight to bring your baby home. As you can see, it's not a "nice to have," but a "must have," in order to have a healthy pregnancy.

❧

I had to drag myself out of bed the next morning. I didn't want to go see Dr. Davidson. I didn't want to have the ultrasound that I was certain would show we'd lost the baby.

The irony wasn't lost on me, either. Prior to the bleeding, I had already developed a pregnancy complication: ovarian hyperstimulation syndrome (OHSS), a rare side effect of IVF. My belly was huge and filled with fluid that had already been drained a few times by an extremely large needle that should not go anywhere near where it needs to go.

I looked like I was five months pregnant, yet we were walking into a fertility clinic to see if there was actually a baby with a heartbeat.

Within minutes of waiting, I was situated in the exam room, and we waited in silence for my doctor to come. I noticed a picture of a woman's reproductive system with all of its parts labeled. If I could have shot lasers from my eye to blow that picture up, I would have.

Why can't my insides look like that? Organs perfectly in their place, unaffected by disease. Actually working properly so I could get pregnant and stay pregnant easily. My very lazy, inept, broken uterus can't seem to get any of this right. . . .

In the middle of my uterine rant came a soft knock on the door.

Sonil and I squeezed our hands together as Dr. Davidson walked through the door, followed by a nurse. He had a somber look on his face as he greeted us and got the machine ready for the ultrasound.

I had had dozens upon dozens of ultrasounds with him prior to this moment, some for pain management and many more for each round of fertility treatment. Since my very first one, I'd tried to read his face while he was performing an ultrasound. I would look intently for any furrow of his brow, a twitch of a lip to see if I could make sense of what he was seeing before he told me so I could brace myself for whatever came next. Every time, I got nothing. The man has an excellent poker face.

He had been quiet for what felt like several minutes. He hadn't even said a word. Dread set in. It had to be bad news.

Eventually, I closed my eyes. The longer he took, the longer we pushed out the inevitable heartbreak. The longer that happened, the more I sat in my anxiety, feeling miserable. Waiting for test results is like that: You feel helpless, because you know whatever's happened has already happened. It's a matter of whether you want to know or what the problem is.

Just as my eyes shut to the darkness, I heard what sounded like horses running through the field. My eyes flew open and I stared at the ceiling, trying to make sense of that unfamiliar sound.

"That's the heartbeat," Dr. Davidson said with a smile.

I freaked out. "*My* heartbeat?! Why's it beating so fast??" I knew I was anxious but this did not sound right.

He laughed and turned the monitor to show me.

"No. It's your baby's heartbeat. Congratulations!"

The hamster wheel in my mind froze as I took in the thunderous claps of this tiny bean's very first organ.

My body is carrying a baby that has a heartbeat?! How did this happen?

Sonil and I were laughing in bewilderment, and we couldn't take our eyes off of the screen. There was a real baby in there with a real heartbeat. We were shocked and so relieved.

Sorry, body, for all the horrible things I said to you over the last 24 hours. High-five, uterus—you're actually doing it!

We breathed out so much of the fear and worry we had been holding in for the previous 24 hours and felt physically lighter as the weight lifted from our shoulders.

But the question still remained: What was going on that was making me bleed so much?

Dr. Davidson showed me again on the monitor complication #2: a subchorionic hematoma (SCH).[11] A subchorionic hematoma (or subchorionic hemorrhage) is a very common complication during pregnancy in which a part of the chorionic membranes, which surround the embryo and amniotic sac, tear away from the uterine wall. This tear and the clot that comes from healing that tear can cause bleeding. It usually resolves itself before the second trimester and is typically monitored just in case it's impacting the course of the pregnancy.

"Okay, so this is something new, not the OHSS?" my husband asked.

I felt the weight on my shoulders again. Of course it was something new. Why wouldn't it be something new? I took back my high-five from my uterus. *We are not friends..*

I didn't care that it's a common complication after IVF and that it happens to many women. You know what else is common? Mice in New York City apartments. Mosquito bites in tropical countries. Pneumonia!

It being common did *not* make me feel better. Add that onto the fact that this was complication #2 in the first six weeks of pregnancy, and I was not amused. This sounded like really bad news, and the hamster wheel was spinning faster than ever before.

Dr. Davidson could see I was worried still. He reassured us that it was small and he had seen hundreds of cases in which this resolved itself by the end of the first trimester. He acknowledged my anxiety, without saying "Don't worry" (the two most useless words in situations like these), and reminded me that he was available and to call or email if I had any questions at any time.

I was terrified but the reassurance that he was there for us helped me breathe a bit easier. It reminded me, again, we weren't alone in this and he was there for us no matter what happened. I trusted that he wouldn't be annoyed if I called later that day or every day until the end of first trimester. I knew that he would take my worries seriously, even if data and professional experience showed him that we would be okay.

We went home feeling a mix of emotions: Worried about what could happen but trusting that if anything did happen, Dr. Davidson would be by our side helping us to figure it out as quickly as possible. We slept that night hoping to wake up to a better day.

The next morning, I had another large bleed. I had so many giant clots it would have concerned my gynecologist if they had happened during a regular period pre-pregnancy. I was panicking. My body felt tight. My brain was going a million miles a minute.

I called Dr. Davidson again. I needed him to be looped in, to hear some reassurance and create a plan. A plan is exactly what I got. "If you want to do everything you can to stay pregnant, I suggest you stop working"—words I will never forget him saying to me.

He reiterated that if I was going to miscarry there was nothing we were going to be able to do about it, but if this was just the hematoma acting up, then my restricted activity levels should help.

He told me to put my feet up, take a load off, take a break, and wait to see what would happen.

Roger that.

I trusted him and I listened to my body. Rest sounded like just what my needed.

My mind slowed down. I put my feet up. I slowed down. I forced myself to breathe feeling hopeful that the bleeding will stop and we'd soon enter calm waters in this pregnancy.

Turned out, the bleeding went on for many weeks, which led me back to Dr. Davidson once, if not twice, a week to see what was going on. After every huge bleed, I was sure I had lost the baby.

I'd lie on the exam table, barely breathing, waiting for him to give me the bad news. My brain was rapid-firing all the horrible scenarios in my head and I felt ragged from the fear that I wasn't going to bring this baby home and anger that my body couldn't keep this baby safe, either.

Every time, he (or his partner), would turn the screen toward me and I'd see a bouncing bean with stubby arms and legs and a giant head doing somersaults. I'd have tears in my eyes out of relief and I could feel my entire body relax as I noticed myself taking in air again. My heart rate dropped significantly and I felt a general sense of calm and hope.

In those moments, I attributed the relief from seeing my baby still growing and thriving. It wasn't until I was discharged from the fertility clinic that I realized how much of the relief was from knowing I had a caring doctor who trusted me and supported me through all of the ups and downs. I felt like I had a safety net under me because he believed me every time I told him something was wrong, and he was always there to tweak the plan, strategize, and think outside the box if necessary to help me stay pregnant.

After experiencing such a nurturing, supportive relationship with a doctor like Dr. Davidson, I knew going forward I would expect nothing else from anyone on my medical team.

The decision to choose more doctors to join my team, my village, who were as trusting, caring, and optimistic as he was, was the best decision I made during my pregnancy. As the number of complications grew throughout my pregnancy, I visited my OB and high-risk OB (also known as a maternal-fetal medicine specialist [MFM] or a perinatologist) more and more frequently. Seeing them, speaking with them, and discussing my concerns translated to changes my body. When I saw my MFM, contractions slowed for hours after the appointment. My heart rate stayed down. Aches and pains improved. I slept better that night.

None of my doctors lied to me, gave me false hope, or sugar-coated the truth. They were all very open, honest, and direct with me. We had difficult conversations about some of the hardest things a parent-to-be can hear: termination, hospitalization, prematurity, fetal demise, among others. But I felt these positive physical changes after every single appointment, whether it ended with good news or a difficult conversation simply because I knew I was in good hands.

My OB and MFM cared about me and my baby. They trusted me and my concerns. They helped me feel like we were all one big team on this journey together. Never once did I feel alone or like I had to figure it out on my own. Never once did I feel like they didn't believe me when a new problem arose. At the time, I didn't realize how invaluable and critical this was to the course of my pregnancy, my health, and the health of my baby.

🌿

As I was doing research for this book, I came across countless resources that showed how imperative a close, supportive doctor-patient relationship is and how important a doctor's belief in a positive prognosis is on your health. The more I read about it, the more I wanted to shout it from the rooftops, because this is a part of your high-risk pregnancy experience and stress management plan that you have full control over.

A strong, supportive, optimistic doctor-patient relationship is not just important for emotional support. It is an essential aspect of your prenatal care, especially if you're going through a high-risk pregnancy because of its impact on your stress response and the resulting changes to your hormonal, immune, and nervous systems.

So how can you make sure you have a trusting and nurturing medical team in place that's conducive to helping you have a healthy pregnancy? Here are some questions to ask yourself:

☐ Does my doctor trust my instincts?

☐ Does my doctor view us as partners, working together to give me the best chance possible at a long, healthy pregnancy?

☐ Does my doctor view my health complications as a challenge that can be addressed or a fate etched in stone?

☐ Does my doctor believe that the treatment (or lack of treatment) will work for me or has a chance of working for me?

☐ Does my doctor share the realities of my complication with optimism?

☐ Do I feel hopeful after leaving my doctor's office, even if I received bad news?

☐ Is my doctor present and focused on me and my concerns during my appointments?

☐ Does my doctor value the impact my stress has on the health of this pregnancy?

If you answered *no* to any of these questions, it's time to reevaluate your relationship with your doctor and consider finding another physician who can better support you during your pregnancy.

The most important question to ask yourself is: *How does my body feel after an appointment or conversation with my doctor?*

Your body will show you symptoms of stress even if you feel justified in your head to continue seeing this particular physician. So pay attention to your body. Do you feel more physically relaxed after an appointment? Do you feel an improvement in your symptoms if you have an existing health condition? Do you generally feel "better" physically after seeing or speaking with your doctor?

If you answered *no* to any of those questions, it's time to reevaluate your relationship with your OB or MFM. You're already under tremendous stress worrying about the health and safety of your baby because you're going through a high-risk pregnancy. Under so much stress, your body is not well-equipped to heal or repair the health complication you're facing, nor is it allowing for the medical treatment you're under to be as effective as it could be.

With a positive, optimistic, nurturing, loving, supportive

relationship with your doctor, who trusts you and views you as an equal member of the team and who sees your complications as a challenge that can be overcome (instead of a "doom and gloom" situation that has no hope), positive physiological changes happen in your body. The relaxation response is kicked on, medical treatments work more effectively, and your body is focused fully on doing what it does best: repairing the damage caused by stress, lowering blood pressure, stabilizing glucose levels, and calming smooth muscles like your uterus, so you can stay pregnant as long as possible.

It's not magic. It's not just in your head. It's biology.

CHAPTER 3

The Antidote to Anxiety

*Don't let your mind bully your body into believing
it must carry the burden of its worries.*

—ASTRID ALAUDA

The idea that anxiety can impact pregnancy health and birth outcomes is a difficult pill to swallow for women and for many medical providers. For many, it implies that you, as the pregnant woman, are fully and completely in charge of what happens during your pregnancy and that any complications that you develop are your fault. This is 100% not true.

For many, it also implies effective anxiety management and traditional prenatal care are mutually exclusive—that you either treat your pregnancy holistically or with Western medicine. This is also 100% not true.

As you saw in Chapter 2, having a nurturing, optimistic, and supportive medical team is critical for a healthy pregnancy. In this chapter you'll see why a strong medical team, while essential and necessary, is not enough to help you have a healthy high-risk pregnancy (even if you have complications) and why effective anxiety management is just as critical to your health and the health of your baby.

❦

During a workshop I attended several years ago, the facilitator asked us to make a list of who we are as a way to help us see how we identify ourselves. After we had completed that exercise, he asked us to make a list of characteristics we believe do *not* define us, nor that we identify with.

The first word on my list was *anxious.*

Never in my life had I been consumed by anxiety. Low mood, helplessness, not feeling motivated? Absolutely. But not anxious. In fact, in the face of a crisis is when I thrived. Some of my strongest moments during my graduate training in clinical psychology came when I was in triage mode:

Calling Child Protective Services

Talking to the police

Making a crisis management plan for a suicidal client

When faced with chaos and fear, my senses sharpened. I could think clearly, make a plan, and execute. Sure, I had moments of nervousness. I had plenty of opportunities in life to feel worried, like when my mom was coming back from a major medical appointment or when I had to take the stage for my first solo three-hour dance performance.

But during a health crisis, I owned anxiety. That was true until this pregnancy.

The bleeds became more and more frequent. I passed larger and larger clots. As if that wasn't enough, I developed several more complications. Anxiety and I went from being acquaintances to becoming bosom buddies. My heart was constantly racing. My mouth was frequently dry. My mind was always filled with "what ifs" and questions that had no answers.

I had transitioned from Dr. Davidson's care to Dr. Edwards, a new-to-me OB. After one appointment with her, it was clear I was going to need specialized support so she referred me to Dr. Kim, my MFM.

Dr. Kim was great. She reassured me frequently and gave me hope about the future even though complications were piling on almost weekly. But there was a lot of "wait and see" prescribed to me. I appreciated her conservative approach to my pregnancy, not wanting to do anything drastic or invasive until it was absolutely necessary, but waiting was not good for my Type A+ personality.

I channeled the anxiety into research, trying to convince myself that this was the most productive use of my time and energy.

Dynamic cervix.

Dynamic cervix prognosis.

Dynamic cervix prognosis second trimester.

Dynamic cervix prognosis second trimester after IVF.

Dynamic cervix prognosis second trimester after IVF with subchorionic hematoma.

I'd read everything I could on the Mayo Clinic, WebMD, and PubMed websites without nearly enough answers. I checked online forums for stories from women who had lived through what I was going through. (Turns out there weren't a whole lot, or, at least, not a lot who wanted to talk about it publicly. And the stories that were shared were *scary*.)

Every morning, I'd turn on my laptop with a new search phrase I wanted to ask Google about. I found authors and researchers who specialized in my complications and tracked down every single published piece of literature I could find.

The Google searches had gotten out of control. It had become an addiction. I knew it wasn't good for me so I tried to implement Internet timeouts. One hour of searching, followed by one hour of any other activity that had nothing to do with my pregnancy.

I binge-watched *Desperate Housewives.* Food Network was a loyal companion. Any Hugh Jackman movie was always welcome.

But even then, during the Internet blackouts, there was still a little part of my brain making a list of all the things I had to research as soon as the movie was over. There was never a break. It was clear that even when I was trying to rest, my mind was going nonstop and that tension was feeding right back into my body. Physically resting was doing nothing to turn off my stress response.[1]

Eventually, I had searched so much on Google and PubMed that there was literally nothing new to read. Pages and pages of searches yielded nothing that I hadn't already printed out and reviewed.

Great job, self. You have officially reached the end of the Internet.

My frustration turned into being short with Sonil, snapping at him when he couldn't read my mind about what I needed or making a snippy comment about how lucky he was that he could still walk or go to work (when I knew all he wanted was a break from carrying the load of life on his shoulders).

I couldn't help it.

Not having answers—not having anything to do but wait—pushed me to my limits and at times turned me into someone I didn't recognize. If I could just get some concrete answers, I was sure this would get better.

So I turned to the only resource left that I hadn't consulted yet: The Magic 8 Ball.

Will my baby be okay? I typed into the online version of the game.

That I found an online website for the Magic 8 Ball should have been sign enough that I'd gone off the deep end. That I had asked it a question about my *baby* should have been red flags with sirens that I needed help with my anxiety.

But no.

I waited for the answer anyway. I knew it was ludicrous. I didn't even believe in signs, horoscopes, or psychics—or Magic 8 Balls! But the anxiety had robbed me of any feelings of control over my pregnancy. I needed someone (or something else!) to tell me it would be okay. I hoped against all hope that this could be the positive sign I needed and I could finally calm down.

A few seconds later, the answer popped up.

Better not tell you now.

I felt fire shoot out of my ears.

Better not tell you now?! *ARE YOU KIDDING ME!?! I HATE YOU, YOU PIECE OF GARBAGE!!*

I actually yelled at my laptop as if it were a real person whose feelings I could hurt.

That finally got my attention.

The tears were burning my eyes in rage and frustration. Was I actually angry at the *online Magic 8 Ball* for not comforting me about my baby's prognosis? What happened to me? The person who used to have clarity in the middle of crises, the one who was always calmest and most reliable to make decisions, especially medical decisions. Who was this crazy person that had taken her place?

It was a miracle we'd made it as far as we had in the pregnancy. I was constantly in and out of the doctor's office because bleeds were so huge or something would feel off and I'd want reassurance. Every time the doctor du jour from the group practice told me everything was fine, I'd start looking for clues that they were lying.

"She's not telling me the whole story," I told Sonil one afternoon as I was frantically Googling after another relatively positive appointment with Dr. Kim.

My fingers were flying across the keyboard, and I had 10 different tabs open for 10 different literature searches.

"What are you talking about?" he asked. "Who isn't telling you the whole story?"

Dr. Kim was fantastic. She was very patient with me and I trusted her wholeheartedly. But my anxiety convinced me she was hiding something. *Maybe the prognosis is so bad she doesn't want me to be burdened by it. Maybe she's trying to protect me from additional stress.*

I had a hard time believing that there was *so* much that was unknown about high-risk pregnancies. We're in the second decade of the 21st century, for goodness sake! Why were "wait and see" and "I don't know" more common answers to my questions than actual answers?

So I decided the only reasonable conclusion was she was hiding something. I had gone from being merely anxious during my pregnancy to being flat-out paranoid and totally suspicious.

Seriously, who was I anymore?

I hated this person I had become, who felt so out of control and frustrated all the time. I didn't want those thoughts clouding my mind—the thoughts of all the horrible things that could happen.

I wanted the self-induced fear mongering in my head to stop. I wanted to relax. I wanted to enjoy this pregnancy we had fought so hard for. I wanted to be at peace. For the sake of my sanity and for the sake of the health of my pregnancy, something had to change. Trying to change my thoughts and control the worry wasn't working and it finally occurred to me: I was going about it all wrong.

🍃

Almost all of my clients come to me with a similar experience, telling me that they've never struggled with anxiety in the past. They're Type A, they love to be in control, they love to plan. They're on top of their life. Anxiety is unfamiliar to them.

Then, they find themselves going through a high-risk pregnancy and all of a sudden their anxiety reaches levels they've never experienced in their lives. They have trouble sleeping because the hamster wheel in their head picks up steam as the house gets quiet. They're scared the aches and pains are signs something's wrong with their body or the pregnancy. They become hyper-aware of the shifts and changes happening in their body. The "what ifs" are relentless, as they imagine every possible worst-case scenario. They can't concentrate at work even though they're craving the distraction. They jump every time their phone rings thinking it might be their OB with more bad news. They obsessively Google everything they can think of even though they know it's not good for their sanity. They worry something is wrong with them that they've suddenly become so anxious. That worry spirals into "What if this anxiety is hurting the baby?"

As a pregnant woman, you are responsible for the safety and well-being of a new life, and it's only natural to wonder and doubt if the decisions you're making or the emotion you're feeling are impacting your pregnancy or your baby. However, nature has given you the tools to help you do that to the best of your ability. For example, you've probably developed a "bloodhound nose" to alert you more quickly about dangerous smells in the air or a heightened aversion to certain foods. Anxiety during pregnancy is another manifestation of that protective mechanism because it keeps you risk-averse and on alert, an essential quality when you're responsible for someone else's life.

A mild elevation of anxiety or alertness that does not impact your daily life is to be expected during pregnancy and is unlikely to impact your health or your baby. How do you know if your anxiety is mild or not? Ask yourself the following questions:

- ☐ Am I staying awake at night because I can't relax? Or do I have trouble falling asleep when I do wake up in the middle of the night?
- ☐ Am I running through "what ifs" in my head frequently throughout my day?
- ☐ Have I been moodier and snappier lately, more than I think I should be, despite hormonal changes?
- ☐ Do I feel paranoid or am I always waiting for the other shoe to drop?
- ☐ Is there something in the back of my head telling me my anxiety is too high?

If you answered *yes* to one of the questions above, that's your clue that managing your anxiety is important for your pregnancy health.

The first step in effectively reducing anxiety during a high-risk pregnancy is being able to distinguish it from fear. We use the words interchangeably but psychologically (and even physiologically) the emotions are very different.

Anxiety is a tricky emotion because it lies but it tries to convince you it's telling the truth. Anxiety is a future-focused emotion, so it's not responding to a real threat that exists in the present, but to a potential threat that could exist in the future. For example, a friend of mine was told she'd likely need to be induced for delivery even though she was weeks away from her due date. She could feel her stress response turn on as her shoulders clenched and she began breathing faster. Her body was responding as if there was a threat against her life in that very moment when in fact nothing had changed in her pregnancy or her life.

Fear, on the other hand, is a present-focused emotion that alerts you to a problem *right now*.[2] The best way to tell the difference between anxiety and fear is to understand it in the form of an analogy of traveling on an airplane. Imagine someone who feels anxious about flying. They're nervous on the plane, gripping the armrest tightly and breathing fast because they're worried about what could happen to the plane. They imagine worst-case scenarios like the plane crashing or catching on fire or the engines failing, none of which has happened yet.

Now, imagine a person on the same plane but whose engine *has* stopped working or a plane that *has* caught on fire and is on the way down. This person is not worried about what could happen to the plane. This person is afraid of what is happening this moment.

Unless you are in an imminent medical crisis this minute (for example, rushing to the hospital because you lost your mucus plug preterm or your water broke and you're not near your due date), the fear you feel is not actually fear but rather anxiety. Your brain is screaming at you that your life is in danger right this minute, you're being chased by a bear right now, when you're actually not. Your body's focus becomes purely to keep you safe and the priority to heal and repair your body goes out the window.

The good news is that because most often the fear we feel is actually anxiety, it is in your control to be able to release in order to turn down your stress response so your body can restore functioning to your immune, endocrine, and nervous systems to help you stay pregnant. To do that requires you to get out of your head and into your body. You've heard me say it already and I'll keep saying it throughout the book: We can talk ourselves in and out of anything, but our body never lies. This is why my clients and I rarely spend time using cognitive strategies to change their thoughts (and why I have not focused on cognitive tools for you to try in this book's appendices). They take too long work, they're not a long-term strategy, and they don't address your biggest concern: how to keep your baby safe during your pregnancy.

You are a mama bear trying to protect your cub. Waiting around, not having a plan, feeling like all you can do is sit on your hands is breeding ground for anxiety even if you've never experienced anxiety in your life. Taking a cognitive approach to anxiety management, while very helpful in most other situations, often adds fuel to the anxiety fire during pregnancy. Many of my clients share that they had worked with cognitive-behavioral therapists in the past but during pregnancy the strategies just didn't work nearly as effectively and they didn't understand why.

This happens because the anxiety triggers are mostly physical during pregnancy. Yes, negative thoughts and constant "what ifs" do occur, but the trigger is rooted in your body, not your mind. That's why even if you are able to get their head into a positive, optimistic space, the minute you feel a pain, a pull, or a twinge, all that cognitive work is unraveled and the anxiety is exactly where it was before.

What's worse is my clients share they felt demoralized that so much hard work could be undone in just a few moments, which fed into their existing feelings of helplessness and that their body (and brain) was going rogue and there was nothing they could do about it. Managing your thoughts for pregnancy anxiety is like putting a Band-Aid on a broken leg. Will it stop the bleeding for a while? Maybe. But it won't actually help you the way you need.

The solution, then, is to forget about what's going on in your head and turn your attention to your body. Where is your anxiety showing up for you in your body? How is it presenting itself physically? Try it right now. Pull out a paper and write down all of the physical sensations you experience when you know your anxiety is high.

For example, many of my clients' anxiety presents as preterm contractions. We know it's anxiety-related because when they're able to activate the relaxation response, their contractions slow or stop. For others, anxiety shows up as headaches, body aches and pains, poor sleep, heart palpitations, high blood pressure, or wonky blood glucose readings. It doesn't matter what's going on in their head. Chemical balance has been impacted by the stress response and needs to be restored for symptom management and a healthy pregnancy.

Wherever and however your anxiety presents physically, stay closely attuned to these parts of your body. The success of any anxiety-management strategy is not going to show up as positive thoughts but will show up as a relief of these physical symptoms. That's when you know your anxiety is *actually* being managed properly in a way that's creating positive changes for your pregnancy health. Changes to your thoughts and mood will follow.

The beauty of addressing anxiety by focusing on your body instead of your thoughts is that your attention shifts to achieving relief for a particular symptom (for example, reducing headaches) and the actions you take are very goal-oriented. Making this shift in how you understand, experience, and address anxiety is extremely powerful because it restores a sense of control during a time when you're feeling so helpless.

I realized this during my own high-risk pregnancy and it completely changed the way that I approached my anxiety. I stopped trusting my thoughts and focused solely on my body, knowing that if I could calm my body down, my anxiety would follow.

Most of us grow up believing that our bodies aren't in our control, and that external factors like medicine, doctors, or alternative medicine strategies are required to help us heal from whatever we're inflicted with. We believe that we have no influence on how our bodies heal from wounds, injuries, and health complications. Throughout my life, I was always uncomfortable with how much power we assigned to something outside of us—doctors, medications, treatments—assuming we had absolutely no power at all. When I became pregnant, I completely refused to believe I had no influence on my health—that my pregnancy and baby's life were in the hands of Western medicine and luck and nothing else.

Yes, your body changes so much when you're pregnant. Your body suddenly starts doing things it never did before. Your size and shape change, your digestion goes off-roading, your skin might suddenly look like your 14-year-old neighbor's, and there is suddenly hair in places where there was never hair before! (If that hasn't happened to you yet, you're welcome for the head's up.)

You're suddenly more tired than you used to be, so your productivity declines—and then you beat yourself up for wanting to nap over meeting work deadlines or taking care of others.

You don't recognize yourself anymore and it's confusing! The constant barrage of messages to pregnant women that there's only so much you can do—that during pregnancy your hands are tied and you just have to wait until you get your body back—fuel the notion that you're helpless, which creates and exacerbates anxiety. Best-selling author and OB/GYN Dr. Lissa Rankin says it perfectly: "As adults, we wind up believing we are powerless to control the outcomes of our health, when really we are infinitely powerful."[3]

Once we've accepted that, though, there's still one more roadblock that we run into: the common perception that wanting to be in control is a bad thing.

Look at the language we use to describe people who like to be in control:

Control freak.
Obsessive.
Inflexible.
Tyrant.
Bossy.

The moment we stop judging control as a bad thing and give ourselves permission to accept that we can influence our health, even during a high-risk pregnancy, tremendous changes happen both emotionally and physically.

Our bodies are designed to figure out how to function optimally no matter the circumstances. Biologically, our bodies are always searching for homeostasis, a quiet sea where boats don't rock and where your body works the way it's supposed to. This is absolutely true during pregnancy as well (even if you have pregnancy complications), when your body is always trying to restore that delicate balance among the endocrine, immune, and nervous systems to help you have a healthy pregnancy.

Medicine, technology, and science have found a way to enhance and improve what our bodies know how to do naturally. For example, did you know your heart can create its own bypass when arteries are blocked?[4] If one lung gives out, the other picks up the slack. Same with the kidneys. It blows me away to be reminded of how much our bodies are capable of especially when life is at stake.

Here's an example that's more likely to have happened to you: getting a papercut. You don't *need* a Band-Aid or antibacterial cream to heal from the cut. Your body knows exactly what to do to stop the bleeding, prevent it from being infected, close the wound, and regrow skin so it looks as good as new. Medical advancements like Band-Aids and creams help enhance this built-in protective mechanism for example to fight off infection, but their role is to essentially help our bodies do what they're already naturally built to do: heal.

The same thing is happening during pregnancy. Your body is working overtime to maintain that delicate balance among the immune, endocrine, and nervous systems to help you have a healthy pregnancy. It is *always* striving for that, no matter how broken you feel your body is. The problem is, anxiety, and the resulting stress response, throw these systems out of balance, increasing your risk of preterm contractions and preterm birth by speeding up your "placental clock."[5] Anxiety, stress, and fear also increase your risk of complications such as gestational diabetes, preeclampsia, reduced blood flow to the baby, and infection, which is dangerous for you and baby.[6] Does your anxiety cause these complications? No. But the stress response that's triggered by anxiety does create biochemical changes in your body that translate to an increased risk of pregnancy complications.

This is not to say we should go back to the caveman days and just let our bodies do what's natural, forgetting about medical interventions. The mind-body connection and medical treatment are not mutually exclusive. Sometimes, medical intervention is required because our bodies have been injured in such a way that healing is not possible without assistance (like in the case of a broken arm that requires surgery). Still, these medical interventions enhance and speed up the healing process that our bodies are already naturally engaged in.

There are a lot of scary statistics when you look into all the ways that anxiety can impact your pregnancy health. Medications and medical interventions alone will not suffice and neither will "wait and see." A combination of anxiety management (by way of improving your physical symptoms of anxiety) and medical treatments is necessary to help you stay pregnant as long as possible, even if you have complications.

🌿

One day early in the second trimester, I had a moment that would change the way I'd experience the rest of my pregnancy. It was a warm summer and the sun was beating down on my shoulders as I sat on the sofa, making my butt imprint more and more permanent every day.

I could hear the neighbors through the window scrambling to get their kids out the door for school. Another neighbor was pacing by his window on the phone, complaining to a poor customer service rep who had become his verbal punching bag.

My life had become scenes out of Hitchcock's *Rear Window.*

I was still in pajamas.

I had nowhere to go. No job or colleagues or students or clients expecting me to show up anywhere. So well into the late morning, I'd lounge in my pajamas, trying to kill time for another day that was just like any other.

I was on an Internet timeout but I couldn't find anything on TV to watch that sustained my attention for more than a few minutes.

I felt like an addict in recovery. I wanted to open my laptop. It was sitting right there, next to me. It would only take a second. I could open it and do a quick search. Just one thing. I'd only need five minutes. That's it.

I'll even double my Internet timeout afterward.

I was legitimately negotiating with myself when, out of the blue, I felt a bubbly sensation in my stomach. At first I thought it was my breakfast moving its way through my pregnancy-induced lethargic digestive tract, so I ignored it and went back to watching TV.

It happened again.

And again.

The bubbles came and went with a pattern. A quick Google search led me to the term *quickening*—early signs of movement in pregnancy.

It made me hold my breath. I waited for it to happen again.

Nothing.

I tried talking quietly. Then loudly.

Nothing.

I was just about to unmute the TV that had been on when it happened again.

I squealed!

There was a real, live human in there! That little day 3 embryo had grown so big that I could feel some bubbles of movement. It was communicating with me!

For several moments I froze on the sofa, afraid to move and make it stop. I spoke to the baby and said hi. I introduced myself, as if knowing my name was going to suddenly make it more likely to stick around.

I didn't know what to say but I was ecstatic.

We had made life! A heartbeat was one thing, but movement? The baby was really, really here!

And then the world of reality came crashing down on me like an anvil on Wile E. Coyote. That means there was a real living thing was staying in a house that was causing *a lot* of problems. A real living thing who could lose their life because of my body not being able to get it together.

That made my heart stop.

I became angry, and fierce focus and determined clarity came rushing in. I spoke out loud with no one to hear me but the walls and my floating bean.

"Okay, we need to turn this around!" I said firmly.

I realized I had let go of the reins. I was no longer in control and the helplessness had sent me down the wrong path in my pregnancy. I ranted and complained frequently. I was resentful and angry too often. I was letting circumstances dictate how my pregnancy went and never once stopped to think about how I could impact my pregnancy for the better. Because I thought I couldn't.

Being diagnosed with several complications so early in my pregnancy had sent me flying out of the driver's seat, leaving me feeling like I was being pulled behind a racing car.

Now that there was this little being inside of me that I could feel, it was so abundantly clear how important it was that I was in charge of the pregnancy.

It's my baby. I'm the mom. I'm the protector. As long as I'm alive, this is my job. I get to speak up and ask questions and it is my right to expect answers in return. I get to choose how I want to experience this pregnancy. I get to decide how much stress I let in and how much joy I allow myself to feel.

I said this whole big speech to the empty family room and the bean, who had stopped moving. Had I scared it?

I had no idea how I was going to do this but I knew that I had to.

I closed my eyes and let my mind wander away from the "what ifs" and horrible images of things that could happen to ideas about and solutions for how to make the pregnancy better. I turned away from Google and statistics and back into the clinical training that I had received for so many years prior to this that had prepared me for this day.

It was my crisis, and I could manage it if I wanted to.

I could feel my heart rate rising as I fervently tried to devise a plan. My palms began to sweat as I made a mental list of questions I needed to ask my doctor at my next appointment. I wanted to get up and start organizing the house, making lists of things we needed to make our lives easier because I was *not* going to lose this baby. We were in it for the long haul! I had already been on bed rest (really activity restrictions, not total bed rest) for seven weeks. Let's make it another 27!

I felt my shoulders clench as they do when I'm bracing myself for action. And then I caught my breath. I felt a tightening in my belly. It was not the little fish that was swimming in there. It was way too early for Braxton Hicks contractions, whatever those felt like.

What was *THAT?!*

I had no idea what happened in my body but my instinct was to lie back, close my eyes, and breathe.

So I did.

In. Out. In. Out. Keeping my mind clear. Open. Focusing on the darkness. I felt my shoulders drop and my back relax.

I opened my eyes and all of those plans went out the window. I knew exactly what I needed to do first before everything else. Step 1: Calm down.

I didn't need access to any of my graduate training materials or literature in mind-body integration to know that. I could feel it in my body.

My anxiety was affecting my body and it needed to be handled. Like

"Olivia Pope from season one of *Scandal*" handled. The thoughts, the imaginative worst-case scenarios, the constant chatter about research and statistics and what they all meant made up just one aspect of anxiety. The other aspect was the anxiety that sat in my body.

The one that kept my shoulders tense even when I thought they were relaxed. The one that kept my jaw so tight I woke the following morning in pain. The one that irritated my uterus and later would exacerbate my preterm contractions.

Now don't get me wrong: I knew my anxiety hadn't caused my complications. That's the thing with fertility and pregnancy. There's no *one* thing that causes the complications, physically or mentally. However, there are so many things that impact the pregnancy both physically and mentally quite profoundly and anxiety is one of them.

🌿

The antidote to anxiety and the helplessness you feel is to get back in control. Control, in this case, is a good thing for your health. You want to go from feeling like you're being yanked behind a speeding car to being the driver of the car. It combats helplessness and turns off the stress response while activating the relaxation response, which works to restore the balance of your body systems to help you have a healthy pregnancy.

By taking back control, not only do you feel more powerful and hopeful emotionally, but it has far-reaching consequences in your body. Research has shown that control as a way to manage anxiety and helplessness improves immune function and reduces inflammation in the body,[7] both of which are critical to restoring the healthy balance among the endocrine, immune, and nervous systems that is needed for a healthy pregnancy.

I want to be clear we're not talking about control over the entire pregnancy. No one knows how your pregnancy will end, when it will end, or what will happen to the baby. But I am saying you have control over how you manage your physical symptoms of anxiety and that those changes will translate to physical changes in your pregnancy that will help you manage your complications and stay pregnant.

This not just a personal belief or a theory of mine. It's purely biology.

To start, ask yourself:

Does this sound like something I want *to do, even if I don't know how yet? Do I* want *to shed the helplessness and get back in control of my pregnancy?*

You have to want it and believe in it before any efforts you take will have a chance at impacting your anxiety and your health. If you answer *yes,* you'll be amazed at how many options are available to you to you to help yourself during your pregnancy.

Then ask yourself throughout your day: *What does my body need right now?*

Not what does your mind need. Not what are the swirling thoughts of doom telling you is going to happen. Not giving attention the hamster that won't stop spinning on its wheel. Focus on your body. The goal is not to feel calmer in your head. The goal is to remove the stress that's residing in your body.

Many women reach out to me and tell me that they're trying deep breathing and positive thinking to help themselves stay calm but it's not working. Their anxiety is through the roof and they find temporary relief only for the anxiety escalate again rapidly. They're confused and demoralized, and they don't understand why or what else to do.

Here's why that happens:

When you're worried about the safety of your baby, your body reacts the same way as if you were feeling threatened by a hungry tiger or you thought someone was breaking into your house.

Your physical safety (and that of your baby) is your biggest concern. If someone told you to try deep breathing, positive thinking, or meditation while you are being chased by a bear, would you do it? Probably not. Would it work? Nope. When you're being chased by a bear, your goal is to get to safety. Not breathe deeply or be more positive. It's to be safe.

What that means during your pregnancy is you have to *create* that safety in your body by focusing on your body and giving it exactly what it needs. More rest. More sleep. More water. More food. More muscle relaxation. Whatever it is, you'll only know by asking that one simple question: *What does my body need right now?*

By allowing that question to guide you, instead of paying attention to the other questions and thoughts that are swirling in your head, you're focused on one thing at a time. You set yourself up for success by creating a goal-oriented task that you *can* complete. When you're able to give your body what it needs, you'll feel more in control. As your feelings of control increase, your anxiety will come down. It truly is that simple and powerful.

What's more mind-blowing is what happens next: You'll notice a change to your health. Your preterm contractions will slow, your blood pressure will decrease, your heart rate will stabilize, your pain will dissipate. Everyone experiences these changes differently, but when you do, your experience of your body and what it can and can't do during a high-risk pregnancy will change forever.

A client of mine was on hospital bed rest and her preterm contractions always spiked when she had a session with her therapist. Her nurse became concerned by that obvious pattern and suggested she stop therapy and call me instead because of this mind-body approach that I take. My goal was to stop her preterm contractions regardless of what was going on in her head. I taught her a relaxation exercise that removed all of the tension systematically from her body. What happened next shocked her and her nurse: Her preterm contractions stopped, as could be seen by the monitors, and the negative thoughts also dissipated because her body was telling her brain, "We're safe now." (You can access this guided relaxation exercise at pbres.pregnancybrainbook.com.)

Another woman I worked with came to me because she was experiencing a shortening cervix without feeling any contractions. She had a history of miscarriages and was terrified of losing this baby too. She was scared her anxiety was going to cause a miscarriage. Her doctor said there was nothing she could do but just try to stay calm and hope for the best. She wasn't satisfied with that answer, so she reached out to me. Instead of focusing on all of those negative thoughts, I taught her how to listen to her body, starting with that one very simple question: *What does your body need?*

By doing that, her anxiety came down because she was focused on only one thing: answering that question. As the anxiety decreased, she was able to recognize that she could actually feel the mild contractions that were responsible for her shortening cervix. The sensations had been so mild she couldn't feel them when her anxiety was taking all of her attention. Trusting her body allowed her to give herself exactly what she needed: physical and mental rest, which stopped her contractions and stabilized her cervical length. She went on to deliver at term!

I want to be super clear that anxiety management isn't a cure-all solution for pregnancy complications. It's not going to help fix structural damage or move your placenta away from your cervix, for example. However, it is extremely powerful for managing and even reversing complications that are impacted by stress and the hormonal, immune, and inflammatory changes that the stress causes and it begins with asking yourself one question: *What does my body need?*

Your thoughts aren't the problem. Your thoughts are just a signal your brain is giving you to run and find safety. If you can create that safety in your body, the alarms stop physically and mentally.

The benefit of this one question is long-lasting because it works no matter the circumstance you find yourself in. When your doctor tells you to "wait and see," you know that your body will tell you otherwise. It will tell you when you need more rest, more food, more quiet time, more water. It will always tell you.

Let's pause for a check-in. How are you feeling?

Are you feeling guilty for your anxiety? Are you taking inventory of all the ways that you might have caused the problems in this pregnancy or previous pregnancies? Are you blaming yourself for what's happening? Are you angry at me because you think I'm blaming you?

It's okay if you said *yes* to any of the above.

This is a new way of understanding your pregnancy and it can be really hard to hear. For some reason we've made it seem like anxiety is a fault of ours—that Mom is to be blamed for anything that goes wrong.

Side-eye at Freud.

Take a deep breath.

This is not your fault. Do you know any mother who would not be anxious, worried, and terrified when her baby's life is in danger? It's in our blood to protect our offspring. Your reaction is normal. Your reaction makes sense. Your anxiety is not your fault. Your complications are not your fault. You have to believe that because, until you do, you're going to hold yourself hostage to your anxiety and your guilt.

Give yourself permission to let it go. Show yourself the compassion you'd show your friends. It's okay that you're feeling anxious. Now that you're here, you can do something about it that will help you and your baby in the coming days and weeks.

The question is: Are you ready to do something to bring your anxiety down both mentally and physically? Are you really ready to let go of the security of worrying?

What really changes, though, when you say yes to these questions is really experiencing that you are not helpless during your high-risk pregnancy. You are not as out of control as you feel. You *can* influence the health and trajectory of your pregnancy.

You might still be terrified of losing your baby. You will still be worried about your pregnancy and your baby. That is a fact.

The goal is to help you stay in control despite those anxieties so you can eradicate the helplessness. The goal is for you to realize that you have a built-in repair system that is trying to do exactly what the medical treatments your doctor has recommended are trying to do: help you stay pregnant.

Let's recap.

When you're feeling anxious, ignore your thoughts and focus on what's happening in your body. What are all the ways your body (not your mind) is cluing you in that your anxiety is too high? Pick one symptom and ask yourself what your body needs in that moment to relieve that symptom. Then, give it that.

This goal-oriented, body-centered approach will help you regain control and establish safety, both of which combat anxiety. The ripple effect of all of this, though, is improved health during your pregnancy because you activate the self-repair mechanism that's designed to regain balance in your body and help you stay pregnant. By allowing your body to do what it's trying to do naturally, you will develop a confidence in your body like never before, an awe and a respect for what it is capable of doing (even if you have complications piling up) because you will experience first-hand how hard your body is working to keep your baby inside of you.

That is life-changing.

CHAPTER 4

The Many Faces of Grief

Everyone grieves. Most have forgotten the art of mourning.
Mourning is "going public" with your grief. Excavating the
internal, and pushing it up and out. In a safe space.
Mourning is a path to healing.

—TOM ZUBA

There are so many losses a woman faces when she has trouble
building her family. Miscarriages, ectopic pregnancies, biochemical
pregnancies, stillbirth, and neonatal or infant deaths are certainly
some that come to mind quickly. However, many women who go
through a high-risk pregnancy experience even more losses than
those that result in the end of a life (called non-death losses).[1]

These other types of losses include the loss of health, such as
coping with new medical diagnoses, symptoms of complications,
and even side effects of medications. This loss of health can also
include activity restrictions to help mitigate complications such as
high blood pressure, uterine irritability, or preterm contractions,

which can be especially challenging if you were physically active before pregnancy.

You might feel negatively toward your body or wonder why it's having such a hard time doing something that's seemingly so easy for everyone else around you. You might feel betrayed by your body for not being able to protect your baby the way you had hoped. (We'll explore the associated guilt more deeply in the next chapter.) You might feel like this body isn't yours and this loss of health might result in dissociating yourself from your body, talking about it as if it's an entirely different entity separate from you.

For many who experience a high-risk pregnancy, bed rest or activity restrictions can mean taking time off from work or, worse, termination of employment. This can result in a change in financial stability, which is a tremendous source of stress for women who cannot continue to work during their high-risk pregnancy. The loss of being a financial contributor to your home, and the loss of your identity as an employee, supervisor, or entrepreneur, can trigger tremendous grief (among other emotions of course) which exacerbate the stress response in your body.

Challenges during your pregnancy, especially if you have been recommended to reduce activity, can put a strain on all of your relationships. You might feel a sense of loss that you cannot be physically intimate with your partner or that you can't even connect emotionally because you feel you're both living totally separate lives—you trying to stay pregnant, your partner doing everything else. You might notice that your friendships change. People who you thought would be tremendously helpful and supportive stop calling or visiting, and that loss of support can leave you feeling alone and hurt.

There is also a loss of the dream pregnancy and the blissful ignorance that a positive pregnancy test means a healthy baby in one's arms 40 weeks later. If you're pregnant after fertility treatment or after pregnancy/infant loss, having pregnancy complications can deepen your loss of ignorance. A client once said to me, "I had trouble getting pregnant. The least my body could do is have an easy pregnancy. But no. Everything has to be a fight."

There are so many types of losses that you experience during a high-risk pregnancy, but so few of them are discussed openly. There's an assumption that certain types of loss are valued and acceptable to mourn and others are not. Countless women I speak with tell me they feel like they will be judged for sharing their sadness about any number of losses that didn't result in death, hearing unsupportive and hurtful comments from loved ones about how you should "just be grateful."

This type of advice is tremendously minimizing, not to mention flat-out bad advice. It's based on the assumption that you cannot be grateful and mourn a loss at the same time, and based on the assumption that grieving means you're constantly sad all of the time. This is 100% not true.

It's also based on the assumption that if you simply look away from your grief, it will go away. Unresolved grief is like burying a stick of lit dynamite. It will blow at some time, and the longer you look away from it, the bigger the blow will be. Grief, especially unresolved grief, is a source of stress that is associated with developing physical health complications, especially during pregnancy (as you saw in the Introduction).

As you read this chapter, I encourage you to put aside the urge to quickly switch to positive thinking or to turn away from your grief just because you think someone else might have it worse. I encourage you to allow yourself to honor the losses you've experienced, no matter how trivial they may seem, because your loss is yours and yours alone. You don't have to justify it to anyone.

�($leaf ornament)

Soon after I got married, a family friend invited me to her baby shower. It was hosted at the cutest little restaurant with gorgeous floor-to-ceiling windows that overlooked a quaint garden in the back.

It was the first major event I'd gone to since my wedding so I got to see a lot of friends and family friends who had been there to celebrate our special day. Seeing my friend with her perfect little bump gliding around the room and welcoming her guests gave our mutual friends the opening for the "wink wink, nudge nudge" conversation with me about having children soon. Except Sonil and I already knew it wasn't going to be so easy. We had already had conversations with a couple of doctors who told us that despite being in our 20s our fertility window was small and closing. We also knew we were going to need help to create our family whenever we decided it was time.

Regardless, making babies should never be party chitchat anyway. It ranks up there with cleaning out your navel in public and looking directly at the sun.

Just don't do it.

I was starting to feel suffocated with all of the baby talk. (I know, I know: What did I expect at a baby shower, right?) So I took a walk. I loved the venue and how simple and peaceful it was. But it was the bar that really stood out.

A large, framed portrait, with the mother-to-be and her husband glowing with joy against the warm setting sun, hung in the bar. Her blue and white polka-dot dress perfectly adorned her adorable little belly. The wind was blowing her hair ever so slightly and the love between them was palpable.

That. I want that.

I had never seen a maternity portrait before but I knew I had to do it when I got pregnant . . . if I got pregnant.

Two years later, I was sitting on the sofa in my oversized shirt and the only sweatpants that fit. I hadn't had a haircut in months.

I had been on bed rest for more than eight weeks and was going stir-crazy from not having worked in months. We were almost halfway to my due date and I had already racked up four complications and also discovered we were having a boy. I felt insane from having been cut off from social life. The only in-person contact I had was with Sonil when he came home every night and friends and family when they had time to visit.

My laptop was resting on my legs and I was scrolling through social media trying to keep up with what was going on in the world and others' lives when I saw it: A friend who was due just a couple of months before me had shared the most ethereal photo of herself in a gorgeous white, flowy dress, the sun creating a perfect halo around her and her bump. She looked stunning. Everything about that photo was perfect.

It felt like someone stabbed me in the heart. My eyes burned with tears. I wanted to look away but I couldn't.

Immediately the anger boiled up.

She's SO lucky. She has NO idea how easy she has it.

I couldn't see beyond it. I hated being this person. Resentment made me feel gross, but I felt it like a reflex.

I needed to know I wasn't the only one who felt this way. I reached out to some new friends I'd made during the pregnancy, many of whom were pregnant, some due around the same time. They all validated my emotions, told me stories of when they experienced this type of anger, too, and reminded me that I wasn't alone in feeling this way.

I felt validated.

This emotion sucks and I don't like it but I'm in a unique situation and this is just part of the territory. I'm not usually a resentful person, but right now I'm justified in scoffing at other women's perfect pregnancies.

It didn't bring me the peace I wanted, but it did give me permission to feel how I feel—until someone scoffed at *me*. "At least you're pregnant!" an acquaintance said to me one afternoon while we were Skyping.

It took my breath away.

I felt like she had punched me in the gut and actually knocked the wind out of me. I wanted to retort back with all of the reasons why my pregnancy was not going well. I wanted to make a list of all of the challenges I was facing physically, medically, and emotionally. I wanted to tell her that there was no guarantee this baby was going to come home even though I was pregnant for the moment and that I'd never wish this pregnancy on anyone!

I became defensive, and I shut down. I stopped sharing my feelings about that photo I'd seen and I stopped talking about any of the other emotions that were being stirred up when I heard pregnancy announcements and saw maternity photos online. I decided to keep all feelings to myself, convincing myself it was just better that way.

After a couple of days, I realized the truth to her words. She was right: I *did* have something that she so badly wanted, just like the girl in the photo had something that I wanted badly. I also realized that stuffing my emotions about them didn't feel right either. Even if I wasn't talking about it, I still felt that resentment toward the girl with the photo shoot and all of the other friends who were cropping up on my Facebook feed sharing their pregnancy announcements and their perfect bellies in golden fields.

The *silence* wasn't right. It's not okay for anyone to hide how they are feeling just because things seem worse for someone else.

Better. Worse. They're relative terms. They're not absolutes, but we treat them like they are.

There are always going to be people who have it worse than you or I, and there are always going to be people who have things better than you or I. If we say that we shouldn't feel sad because things can be worse, doesn't that mean we can't be happy because things can always be better?

Ludicrous.

I thought back to that woman who called me out on being

pregnant when she couldn't carry a baby, and I thought about what this must be like for her. She thought of me with my growing midsection, even though I was parked on the sofa with not much of a social life left other than seeing my doctors at least once a week, and she saw what she wanted: a growing belly with a baby. When I saw that woman in the photo, I saw what I wanted: a healthy pregnancy in which I was able to stand up without hurting my baby and an ability to celebrate that.

We both saw things that we wanted so deeply and could not have.

Seeing it through my friend's eyes, it became very clear to me that this resentment and jealousy, and the anger or sarcasm that come with it, are nothing more than a mask for our grief for our losses.

For some reason, though, we've created a culture in which, unless the loss is death, we're not allowed to mourn it publicly. And even then, there's an unspoken time line for how long a parent is allowed to mourn their child publicly before others worry why they're "not over it." What's worse, we've turned mourning into a game in the Pain Olympics. We've started quantifying someone's pain and grief, and pitting it against others', believing it's possible to rank our pain and grief as more or less painful.

When did this become a thing? Why is my pain any worse than her pain? Why is her pain any worse than someone else's pain? What is this desire that we have to box people in and force them to justify their pain and suffering? Isn't it enough that there *is* pain? That there *are* dreams that are being crushed, leaving hearts broken?

The woman club is full of comparisonitis and Pain Olympics. At every step of the way. And it starts so early.

I remember girls in junior high comparing themselves to me to see how much taller they were and feeling good when they surpassed my height.. (Hint: It's not hard to be taller than someone who is just barely above 5 feet tall!) Girls compared notes with each other in college about who sacrificed more food to help them lose weight faster. There was competition about who had a harder time planning their wedding or more challenges with their partner or a more demanding job.

Those very same Pain Olympics carried into the world of infertility and pregnancy: Who has more back pain? Who sleeps the least? Who has more painful shots? Who has worse symptoms from the medications?

Even if there's no one else to compete with, this comparisonitis happens in our heads all the time. We have this entire conversation in our heads—*with ourselves!* We compare ourselves to the stories we know of others, judging ourselves about when it's okay to grieve and when it's not okay, telling ourselves to be positive because this person has it worse or because it could be worse for us right now. The minimizing of grief has become an epidemic.

And we wonder why we can't band together and support each other during the hardest times of our life. Whether that's adolescence or infertility, motherhood or mid-life, we as women need each other, but we turn on each other, and ourselves, so quickly that we don't have a chance to give and receive the support we each deserve. That sense of isolation, lack of support, feeling like you might threaten others around you so you stay quiet for fear of rocking the boat—guess what that does to your body?[2]

Lizard brain. Grizzly bear. Run.

We all have losses in our high-risk pregnancy that we have to grieve. That we deserve to grieve. Some of them may make sense to other people and some may not.

Who cares?

They're you're losses. It's your grief. You don't have to justify to anyone. You are entitled to honor that grief, and you *need* to release it in order to have a healthy pregnancy.

◊

When I realized what was happening, it occurred to me that I had a choice and I chose not to participate in these Pain Olympics. Emotions, experiences, joys and losses, grief and mourning are not a zero-sum game. We can all be hurting at the same time and can join together to heal.

We need to create that space for ourselves and each other. I may not understand your loss or be able to sympathize with it because it may be a loss I wish that I had. And vice versa. But that doesn't mean you should ever feel bad about feeling bad.

My friend was allowed to grieve the fact that her body couldn't maintain a pregnancy as long as mine had. To her, regardless of the complications, she wasn't able to carry a child as far as I had. That loss of her dream of being pregnant, of hopes for her future, of experiencing this, was devastating for her and something she needed to grieve.

Just like that, I needed to grieve the loss of a pregnancy in which my baby and I were safe physically. I had to grieve the loss of going through rites of passages that I wanted to experience to mark this special pregnancy and baby. I had to grieve the loss of the dream pregnancy and even the loss of ignorance that being pregnant automatically means a healthy pregnancy and a baby to bring home. No loss is more justified than the other.

My high-risk pregnancy taught me so much about releasing grief and allowing myself to ride through these feelings without judgment. It also taught me too how to be mindful of who to turn to for support. I would never expect this acquaintance, who couldn't get pregnant, to understand or be able to support me through my grief of the loss of a healthy pregnancy. But I do expect that she respect it and not take out her grief on me through anger or resentment.

And the same expectation goes for me. When I see photos of maternity photo shoots or I see women who are far more physically active than I was during my short pregnancy, or I see families with the number of children that Sonil and I wished we could have, it's my job to recognize that the sarcastic comments, the eye rolls, and the gut punches that I feel are *my* grief. It is my grief trying to get my attention to tell me "We've got more work to do."

It's a life-long process but when pregnant, releasing this grief is critical because avoiding it does impact the health of your pregnancy.

𝕊

Grief is a psychological experience that we feel on an emotional level. However, the resulting stress from this emotion deeply impacts our bodies physically, especially during pregnancy.

Research has shown that unresolved grief during pregnancy is linked to delivering low birthweight babies,[3] preterm delivery,[4] and a 6% increased risk of early-onset preeclampsia.[5] While the exact pathways from grief to pregnancy complications and prematurity are not yet known, what has been shown repeatedly in the literature is how much stress your body is under when you are grieving a loss of any kind.

Cortisol levels (a stress hormone) are high when grieving, which impacts the immune system, reducing its functionality and making you more susceptible to infection[6] and illness. Experiencing grief also affects sleep quality, causing you to wake up more frequently and sleep less deeply.[7] This is even true for women who don't otherwise experience sleep disturbances or don't necessarily feel anxious.

Grief has also been linked to an increase in pro-inflammatory chemicals in the blood. These pro-inflammatory immune cells can wreak havoc on the health of your pregnancy, increasing your risk of numerous complications such as preeclampsia, gestational diabetes, preterm labor and delivery, as well as impaired blood flow to baby and delivering a small for gestational age baby.[8]

What's more, grief and stress (and the resulting physiological and social changes) are both tremendous risk factors for developing depressive symptoms or clinical depression during pregnancy. Antepartum depression, though not discussed nearly as frequently as postpartum depression, also adds risk factors for pregnancy complications. In fact, one study showed that experiencing depressive symptoms during pregnancy (such as persistent low mood, hopelessness or helplessness, etc.) poses a risk for preterm birth and low birthweight babies similar to smoking 10 or more cigarettes per day.[9]

All this to say, managing your grief is so much more than helping you feel happier or cope better. It's essential for you to have a healthy pregnancy, especially if you have complications already. This is absolutely possible to do without delving deep into pain you don't want to feel again.

I worked with a woman who usually slept like a log. Even during pregnancy, she would fall asleep easily, wake up to use the bathroom several times a night, and then fall straight back asleep. She knew something was wrong when she started waking up in the middle of the night and had trouble falling asleep. Her friends counseled her that it was typical for pregnancy and she should "get used to it" before the baby came, but she had a gut feeling something else was going on. When she reached out to me, she reassured me several times that she's not anxious; she doesn't have racing thoughts or the never-ending hamster wheel of "what ifs."

When I delved deeper into what else was happening in her life, she realized that she was fast approaching the due date of the baby she had carried prior to this pregnancy. She had tried to stay so busy that she had forgotten the date consciously, but her subconscious and her body remembered. Her grief was resurfacing in a way she had never imagined, trying to get her attention so it no longer remained unresolved.

When clients reach out to me for bereavement support, after a miscarriage or a non-death loss, most of them ask me, "Am I going to cry every session?" I get why the ask. We have ingrained in us this idea that without pain, we can't make any strides toward healing or success. "No pain, no gain" is an awful adage to live by.

My philosophy is that if you've experienced loss of any kind, you've already been through enough pain. Why make the healing process just as painful? Who needs more pain in their life? I certainly don't! And neither do you.

Gentle grief release starts by recognizing that the grief does not reside nearly as much in our heads as we think. Instead, it hides in our bodies, trying to find a way out. This is why you can feel positive, happy, hopeful, and optimistic; think that you're "over it" only to feel the gut punch of a baby shower invitation that sends you spiraling into an eye-rolling, cursing frenzy; or suddenly burst into tears when you see a pregnant woman walking by showing her perfect bump. This grief—the one that's impacting your mood, immune function, and nervous system—sits deep in your body, trying to get your attention.

Releasing this grief requires first, acknowledging without judgment that it's there. No "I shouldn't be . . ." or "I should. . . ." Remove that "S" word from your vocabulary. No Pain Olympics. Just acknowledge it. Give yourself permission to write it down so it's real and tangible.

I'm sad because I will never experience a vaginal birth.

I'm grieving that despite struggling to get pregnant, now I'm struggling to stay pregnant.

I'm disappointed that I won't have a baby shower.

I'm heartbroken that I need medication during my pregnancy.

Whatever it is, write it down and acknowledge it. Then, make a list of everything you love about yourself.

Here's what I've learned about grief in my years of professional grief counseling, grief and bereavement research, and my personal experience with mourning many losses (death and non-death): The only way to release grief for good is with self-compassion.

You've likely heard that you have to go through the fire to get to the other side. Well, if the fire is grief, compassion is the cloak that will protect you from getting burned.

If you're disappointed in this solution, wishing I had shared some type of Jedi mind trick that will shut the grief switch off, I get it. This was really hard for me to do too. It still is, depending on how deep my grief sits. Sometimes, during my pregnancy, I found it so hard to write anything positive about myself that I cried because it felt like one more thing I couldn't do.

The trick, if you really want one, is that you'll never be able to write this list with your head. It's not meant to be written with your head. Be present in your body and feel where the grief is sitting. Is it a kink in your back? A sinking feeling in your stomach? A headache? Feel it. Acknowledge it. Then from that space, start your list with this sentence:

Even though I'm grieving _____, I am loved.

From there, let the pen flow. Don't think. Just feel and write a list of everything you love about yourself. You'll be amazed what comes out and how comforted you feel by that cloak that's protecting you.

One more thing many of my clients tell me when we're about to start our grief release work is that they're scared of allowing themselves to feel down, to feel sad, to really sit with the heartbreak because they worry if they feel it, they may never be able to come out of it.

We're so afraid of our feelings because we think for some reason that if we feel them, we'll get stuck in them and then they'll start to define us. However, not allowing ourselves to acknowledge our emotions like anger and jealousy, sadness and disappointment, hurts us. Literally. Physically.

Psychology professor Gay Hendricks said it perfectly when he wrote, "When feelings are fully felt, they do not last long at all. It is only when we put on the brakes during the process of experiencing a feeling that it feels endless."[10]

It's okay to mourn the loss, whatever loss, you're grieving.

Feel it.

Own it.

Wrap yourself in compassion.

Release it.

Lather, rinse, repeat.

CHAPTER 5

Escaping Your Personal Prison

If you make someone feel guilty about their mistake, then you have not forgiven them. That guilt is itself punishment.

—SRI SRI RAVI SHANKAR

It seems as if guilt and motherhood are inextricably linked. As if to be a mother requires you to feel guilty about *something* at any given moment. For some, guilt becomes a daily experience starting as early as pregnancy, doubting at every turn if you're doing the right thing for your baby. During a high-risk pregnancy, this guilt is exacerbated for many women because they feeling responsible for their complications and how the complications are impacting, or could impact, the baby's health.

You might feel like a terrible mother because it feels like your body is failing your baby. You might feel like *you're* failing your baby for having extra challenges that pose risks to your health and your baby's health.

This guilt, and that endless chatter in your brain reminding you of the weight of the responsibility on your shoulders (and literally in your belly), sits heavy. It creates a negative feedback loop, impacting your self-esteem, your mood, and your confidence, which perpetuates the feeling of guilt and that you're not doing enough. That *you're* not enough.

Not only that, guilt closes the door on hope and joy, preventing you from enjoying milestones and special moments of your pregnancy. Most concerning, however, is how closely tied guilt is to the physiological stress response that puts you at added risk for pregnancy complications.

The good news is that releasing yourself from the grips of guilt requires a mental shift that you can make as soon as you're ready. Is guilt common during a high-risk pregnancy and motherhood? Yes, but it does not need to hold you hostage nor dictate how you experience your pregnancy or your transition to parenthood.

$$\mathscr{g}$$

In college, I met a lovely girl through my social psychology class who was obsessed with the TV show *Sex and the City*. She had bought all of the DVDs of the series, and one afternoon after a session with our graduate student instructor, she asked me to come for a binge-watching session.

I wasn't up for it. I wanted to study. I always wanted to study. It was my happy place.

"But it's Friday night. Come *ooooon!*"

I knew I should be more social. There were no impending exams or paper deadlines coming up. There was no *real* reason for being cooped up in my apartment other than the fact that I was addicted. To the research and the data. The smell of the library.

Yes. I was that kid.

The internal battle in my head was getting too loud and I needed it to stop so I finally agreed.

"Okay, fine. I'll come."

She gave me her address and ran off to her next class as I walked down the hill toward my apartment.

At about 5 p.m., I walked over to her apartment, which was in a neighborhood I'd never been. It was lined with big, beautiful oak trees and old homes that had been converted into multiple apartment units.

I walked up the steps and knocked on her door, ready to have a fun girls' night in. Instead, I was met with a tear-stained, red face who peeked from a barely cracked open door.

She and her long-distance boyfriend were in the middle of a huge fight on the phone.

"Can we do this another time?"

Of course, I agreed, and turned to leave. She felt terrible about canceling at the last minute, so she sent me home with the Season 1 box set and told me to bring it back to class when I was done.

That night, I popped in the first disc and watched it all the way through. By the end of the weekend I was done. So much for spending time with my books.

Over the course of the semester, I'd burn through a season and bring it back to her during lecture, and then she'd give me the next season to watch. I'd pop it into the CPU of my desktop computer, hearing the whirring of the machinery, and watch while folding laundry or reviewing notes from lecture earlier in the day.

She was so generous, never asking me to return them sooner than I was done. She just reminded me to be careful with them because they were expensive (and her favorite). I took that responsibility on very seriously.

After a few weeks, life had become really hectic. With final exams, papers due, and deadlines for internship applications approaching, my binge-watching had come to an end. My tunnel vision had been restored.

Study. Eat. Class. Study. Eat.

That was my day. Every day. I loved it. But it was busy.

As the end of the semester approached, I handed her back the box set that I had with me, Season 5. I never got to finish it, but she wasn't going to be around for the summer. It had been fun and I thanked her for introducing me to a new show I would not have watched otherwise.

Two years later, as I was clearing out my apartment, ready to move elsewhere in Berkeley for my first job post-graduation, I found a lone DVD, stuffed at the back of my desk.

Sex and the City. Season 5. Disc 2.

Crap!

I had forgotten to put it in the box when I gave it back. And, two years later, I couldn't remember her name or where she lived or how to get it back to her. I felt awful.

How could I do that? I should have checked the box more carefully before giving it back to her! She must be so mad at me for keeping one. Maybe she thinks I did it on purpose. Is that why she never called me back when she returned in the fall? I'm such a bad friend.

In the weeks leading up to graduation, I searched for her on campus.

I kept the DVD safely in a red CD case. Away from dust and scratches. Just in case I ever saw her again.

It was another hot summer day. My favorite season of the year, and I had been cooped up inside the house on bed rest for four months and counting. The novelty of staying at home had worn off weeks ago. I was bored from not working, under-stimulated by being alone most of the days and frustrated with my body for not letting me move as fast as my head was going.

Sonil had started looking exhausted. Between the stress of keeping up with several pregnancy complications and the pressures at work, plus having to shoulder all of the responsibilities at home, he was tired.

My first trimester had been hard because of two complications, but my second trimester, the one that was supposed to be the easy one of the three, was also not looking great, and the stress just kept piling on Sonil's shoulders.

He left for work and I lay my head back on the sofa in defeat. I heard neighbors trying to rush their dogs with their morning business so they could all go back inside. I heard a neighbor who was a nurse at a local hospital running with his keys in his hands. Late again, as always.

Delivery trucks were pulling up, dropping of packages, and heading off. Parents were handing off babies to nannies at the front door as they raced to get to work.

And me. Sitting on the sofa. Staring at the TV. Again. Nowhere to go. Nothing to do. No one expecting me to be anywhere.

I looked at the clock. 8 a.m. If I watched a movie, it would take me to mid-morning. I could have a snack. That would kill 30 minutes.

I'd learned to eat very slowly to pass as much time as possible.

As I did every day, I tried to come up with as many activities as I could to fill up the time that taunted me with its emptiness.

I went through our DVD drawer. I'd already binged on *Friends* and *Gilmore Girls*. I could do *The Office* next. I pulled out the box of DVDs. Right behind it was the red CD case from years ago.

Sex and the City. Season 5. Disc 2.

I opened it slowly to look at it. Still in perfect condition. Still not mine.

I sat down on the floor looking at it, rolling my hand over it, and remembering that sweet girl from so many years ago who trusted me with something that was so important to her.

Trusted *me*. With something *so important*.

I started to feel the tears burn my eyes as I tried to fight them back. I had let her down.

I felt a lump in my throat that I couldn't swallow.

She trusted *me*. She *trusted* me.

My breath was caught in my lungs.

I broke her trust.

And now, Sonil trusts me—and I'm letting him down. This baby, my son, trusts me to keep him safe and I'm failing with that too . . . .

Just like that, the dam burst open and the tears came flooding out, as did the deep, heavy sobs.

Without real words forming in my head, I saw images. Clusters of images flashed one after another.

The bags under Sonil's eyes. The extra gray hairs that had started to grow above his sideburns. How much more slowly he'd walk up the stairs in the evening. His huge eyes that flashed with fear every time I got up to go to the bathroom in the middle of the night. The sigh he let out every week when he brought up the last bag of groceries.

The texts and photos my nonprofit volunteers would send me of the extra time they were all putting in to make sure we kept up with our deadlines and our meetings.

The disappointment in my friends' voices when I had to decline birthday dinners, engagement parties, and wedding invitations.

This little boy who had done nothing wrong and had never asked for such a tumultuous start to its life.

This body that was doing such a terrible job at keeping this little person safe. This body that I was so angry at for betraying me and my baby. This body that was the reason I couldn't help at home. Support my friends and family. Go to work.

This body that kept having problems, that made me sit here at home day after day, not trusting it to get it together.

The tears kept flowing. The sobs kept shaking my body. The images kept coming. The guilt completely took over. I had transformed from a strong, determined (yet bored) pregnant woman to a pile of mush consumed by self-blame.

That's the thing about guilt: It just needs one tiny hole, and then the dam crashes wide open.

I needed that moment, though. I needed to feel it. To think all of these thoughts. To feel the guilt.

Because it was just getting stuffed inside and silenced.

I had tried sharing it with my friends and family before. Sometimes even with Sonil.

"I don't know what I'm doing wrong," I lamented to my best friend.

"I must have done something to deserve this," I said to Sonil and many, many occasions.

My confessions were always met with sad eyes, as my loved ones didn't know how to fix this for me, and were met with comments like "You didn't cause this!" and "This is not your fault!"

I *know* I didn't cause it. I *know* it's not my fault. I didn't *cause* my complications. I know all of this in my head. But I didn't feel it in my heart. I still felt responsible.

"Whose job is it to grow this baby?" I yelled at Sonil through tears one evening after a particularly difficult doctor's appointment.

"Well, yours," he said slowly, followed quickly with "But it's my job to help you. And the doctor's job to take care of you. You're not solely responsible. You're not alone in this fight. It's a team effort."

It didn't feel like a team effort.

The baby was in *my* body. *I* felt the bleeds before anyone else knew about them. *I* felt the contractions before any monitor picked them up. *I* felt the fatigue before any blood test showed a problem.

It was *my* job to grow this embryo into a person that was ready to come into this world. And I felt like I was failing at it every step of the way.

Couldn't get pregnant without help.

Couldn't stay pregnant without help.

The reality cut deep. Platitudes and niceties weren't going to make this any better.

I wiped my tears on the back of my hand, the blurs turning into colors and shapes until I could see clearly again through dry eyes.

Sex and the City. Season 5. Disc 2.

It felt like a lifetime ago, that mistake. And yet holding the DVD case transported me back to that moment as if it were yesterday. Like I didn't want myself to forget.

Like I didn't want myself to forget.

That took a moment to sink in.

I moved myself back over to the sofa, ran my hand over the DVD, and let the feeling pass through. I didn't want myself to forget that I had let her down. I was holding myself hostage to a mistake from more than a decade before, because I felt I deserved it. It sounds ridiculous when you put the subconscious feeling into words, but stick with me.

Keeping the DVD had gone from a practical solution (maybe I'll see her again before graduation) to a symbol of a mistake I didn't want to make again because of how bad I'm sure my actions made her feel.

And yet here I was, almost 10 years later, doing it again. Except this time it's not a DVD. It's words.

It's my *fault.*

I'm *broken.*

My body is *failing* our baby.

They're words that I refused to let go of because it was a lesson to myself. A reminder so that I will never forget. Every emotion serves a purpose. The purpose of holding onto these words, I realized, was to punish myself.

🌱

You might be thinking, "Okay, Parijat. Now you've lost it. No one punishes themselves on purpose."

But we do. We all do. Each and every one of us.

The guilt feels so justified because there's physical proof of problems. *Hey look, I'm bleeding again. Hey look, my contractions are back even though I'm weeks away from my due date. See? I* am *broken.*

You feel like your pregnancy problems are your fault, you internalize the blame, and you feel like there's nothing you can do to make it up to your baby. Those thoughts are powerful and have cascading effects on your physical health because your brain does not know the difference between a negative self-thought, self-disparagement, and being chased by a bear.[1] So, negative thoughts slam on the brakes of your self-repair system and trigger the stress response, which, as you've seen throughout this book, throws off the hormonal, neurological, and immune balance in your body that's necessary to have a healthy pregnancy.

Research has shown that when we feel like we can't do something to make the situation better for what we feel at fault for, we punish ourselves, specifically by denying ourselves pleasure. This has been named the *Dobby Effect.*[2]

You don't ask for the foot rub that you so desperately want because you tell yourself your partner is doing so much already so why add more to their plate? You say no to a friend who offers to come sit with you when you're on bed rest (even though company is exactly what you're craving) because you tell yourself you don't want to burden her (even though *she's* the one who offered). You refuse the last piece of pie even though everyone saved it for you because you don't feel like you deserve it.

Sound familiar?

Psychologically, when we feel guilt, our brains are designed to search for relief because it is such an unpleasant experience. When we say something hurtful to a friend or we forget our partner's birthday, we feel guilty, but then we apologize to repair the relationship. Maybe we even find a way to make up for the transgression, like an extra big gift or scheduling a coffee date. Whatever we do, with words or actions, it ultimately relieves us of the guilt.

However, in the case of a high-risk pregnancy when you didn't actually do anything wrong, you take the blame for it *and* you feel there's nothing you can do to make it up to your baby. So you punish yourself as a way to relieve that guilt. It acts as a way for you to show remorse,[3] to say "I'm sorry" to your partner and your baby without having to say it.

However, it doesn't stop there.

As you can imagine, emotions like guilt are not just unpleasant to experience psychologically. Guilt is a stress-inducing emotion, meaning it causes stress-related changes to your body physiologically, such as lowered immunity and increased inflammation, as seen by elevated pro-inflammatory substances in the blood.[4] In fact, one particular research study found that people who blamed themselves for a traumatic experience that they actually had no responsibility in experiencing had the greatest elevations in proinflammatory substances in their bodies out of all the participants who experienced trauma.[5]

It's not a huge leap to say that when we feel so negatively about ourselves, when we blame ourselves (especially for health conditions we didn't cause), and when we take the responsibility on our shoulders to try and fix it, it's stressful. It takes a toll on your self-esteem and how hopeful you feel about your future, and can set the stage for experiencing depression during pregnancy.

It's a cycle you don't want to get stuck in and it's one that feels hard to break out of until you know how.

♪

In the middle of this eye-opening moment when I realized how I had been punishing myself for so long, I felt another flutter. Stronger this time than before. It could have been an actual hand or a foot.

The baby is getting bigger and stronger. I smiled and put my hand on my belly.

Then it hit me: I was missing it. The guilt was clouding every experience I was having in this pregnancy. It was keeping me from feeling pure, unfiltered joy in moments like this, when my bigger, stronger little MB was punching me from the inside. This guilt was causing me to push people away, leaving me feeling lonely. It was preventing me from truly allowing my body to relax and let it work its magic to help me stay pregnant.

It was my choice what to do. I could buy into the lies that guilt was feeding me, even though they felt *so real*. Sometimes they felt like fact that could never be disputed.

I could choose to keep going down that path.

OR

I could choose to stop punishing myself. I could choose to stop holding myself hostage to this guilt and allow myself to see—and deeply feel—how deserving I was of the love, support, and kindness that I was being showered with. To see that I was deserving of joy, compassion, and peace even though my body was struggling.

I realized that if I didn't make the right choice in that moment, I was going to miss the entire pregnancy. All of it.

Around lunchtime, the one time of day I was allowed to use the stairs, I went to the garbage can in our kitchen, opened it with my foot, held the DVD over it, and apologized.

To my friend from many years ago who introduced me to a TV show that helped me reaffirm my love for New York City.

To myself for holding on to the guilt and punishing myself for so many years and for doing it again now.

And then I threw it away, and with it I felt the guilt melt away.

The time flew by for the rest of the day with a warm feeling in my body, feeling fundamentally changed. Like I'd lifted 250 pounds of weight off my shoulders.

That wasn't the end of my guilt-ridden days by any means. My natural tendency is to take on blame for things I'm not responsible for. Blame and guilt are where my brain goes as default.

But this moment has served as an anchor for me to go back to when I go down those dark, self-punishing paths of taking responsibility for things that I know aren't my fault but feel like they are.

I take the resurgence of guilt as a clue, that there's some healing that needs to be done internally in order to release that guilt. I let myself go there.

I feel it.

Own it.

And then I release it.

Sometimes an episode of *Sex and the City* doesn't hurt, either.

*

Self-punishment happens when we feel we cannot do anything to compensate or make up for the problems we feel we caused—in this case, a high-risk pregnancy that could be impacting the growth and development of your baby. In that very belief resides the solution to releasing guilt: recognizing that it's a choice.

Self-punishment is a choice. Self-blame is a choice. Believing you're powerless to help your baby grow and thrive is a choice.

You know your negative thinking isn't good for you or your health. You know that it's feeding into your low mood and your increasing stress levels. The reason it's so hard to change is because you're not sure what else you *can* do to help your baby, so you default (like I did) to blaming yourself as a way to assuage that guilt, which, as you see now, is harmful to you and your pregnancy.

So, I offer you a different solution to try.

Forget about what's going on in your head—all the negative self-talk, the blame, the names you're calling yourself. We're not going to try to change those because—let's face it—if it was that easy, you would have done it already, right?

Instead, let's focus on what you *can* do, which is to alleviate your physical symptoms of guilt. Think of something in particular that brings up feelings of guilt and self-blame. Maybe it's a complication you have or an ultrasound that showed baby is small for gestational age. Think of one thing that really brings up feeling like this is your fault or you could do better.

Then turn your attention away from those thoughts and toward your body. Where in your body do you feel your guilt? How do you describe that feeling?

I've had clients describe it as a sinking feeling in their stomach or butterflies all over their chest. One woman shared that her throat would become dry every time she felt guilty for having a pregnancy complication. Another shared that she'd get a headache. It's different for everyone, so focus on your particular body. Where do you feel guilt and how would you describe it? Use as many details as you can.

A simple exercise to try when you're ready to release the guilt is to close your eyes and visualize that physical sensation. For example, if it feels like an anvil on your chest, picture it as vividly as you can. With every inhale, keep your focus on the anvil. With every exhale, visualize it lifting up higher and higher. Feel the weight on your chest diminish and disappear.

The goal of this exercise is not to change your thoughts. As you've seen, it has nothing to do with your thoughts. The intention is to notice how much calmer, lighter, and quieter your body feels after you've done it. Our brains don't know the difference between a visualization and a real visual perception so imagining the weight from guilt lifting from your body is tremendously powerful. By turning down the stress response through this visualization, your body and brain will experience a sense of safety again. The threat is gone. You are safe. It is only when you experience safety that you can work on your thoughts, replacing the self-blaming ones with more empowering ones.

One client worked with me because she was feeling guilty for her previous miscarriages, convinced she'd done something to cause them. She had tried positive affirmations and cognitive therapy to no avail. This unreleased guilt then carried over from her past pregnancies into her current pregnancy, where she was facing two health complications. The cumulative effect of the self-blame for the miscarriages and the pregnancy complications came out through her body very strongly. She frequently woke up in the middle of the night and had trouble falling back asleep. She had an elevated heart rate, frequent crying episodes, and tension headaches most days (despite having no history of headaches prior to this pregnancy).

After completing this exercise together, she opened her eyes with tears falling down her face, feeling as if she could breathe again. As she checked her heart rate during our session and for the rest of the day, she was shocked to see how much it had come down and stayed down. That night, she slept through the night, something she hadn't done in months.

These incredible physical changes are possible for you too. The first step must be to establish safety in your body, which is done by releasing the guilt that's trapped inside. Visualizations are powerful tools that can help with the release of strong emotions like guilt, their effectiveness evident in symptom relief in your body. The stress from holding onto guilt impacts your health but the release can set the stage for repair, healing, and a healthier pregnancy.

CHAPTER 6

The Voice that Never Lies

"It is amazing how many hints and guides and intuitions
for living come to the sensitive person who has
ears to hear what his body is saying."

—ROLLO MAY

It's no secret that in the United States, the healthcare system is far from perfect. Sadly, our medical system in the U.S. has flaws that reach far, wide, and deep. This is especially true when we look at condition of prenatal care.

The United States having one of the highest mortality rates in the world of women during and after delivery is not an accolade anyone is proud of.[1] This fact is made worse by research from the CDC Foundation that concluded that nearly 60% of these deaths are preventable.[2] Not included in these statistics are what are called "near-misses"—women who came close to dying due to a complication from pregnancy or delivery but thankfully survived. About 65,000 women per year fall into this category.[3]

Serena Williams, one of the strongest female tennis players of all time, spoke up about her near-miss experience: a blood clot in her lung that was almost missed by the medical team because the ultrasound came back clear. No amount of fame, fortune, or professional success makes a woman immune to the troubles of our healthcare system.

Medical errors and flaws in the system extend beyond the delivery room, though. Research conducted in 2005 found that more than one-third of doctors failed to ask what was wrong within the first five minutes of the appointment when a patient came in with a concern.[4] As you can expect, identifying the problem and treating the patients' concerns are much less likely in this scenario than when a doctor inquires about the concern immediately.

The challenges of the medical care system run even deeper than these obvious situations, some I'm certain you have experienced yourself. I have had countless clients complain to me about how rushed they feel in the doctor's office or share their frustration that their doctor isn't taking their concerns seriously. These doctors, who are often otherwise very nice, kind, loving professionals, just don't have the time or the resources to provide the patient what she needs.

A client shared recently that she was worried about her baby but she didn't think her OB would take her worries seriously, so she didn't bring up her concerns during her appointments. It infuriated me to hear how the system facilitated a dynamic between physician and patient in which she felt silenced or unsupported.

While we could dedicate an entire book (many have been already written) on the flaws of the medical care system and how much it costs in terms of money, health complications, and lives, the reality is that the system will only change in response to us, as patients, forcing it to change. In this chapter, I walk you through how *you* can navigate through this broken system and receive the medical care you and your baby need. You deserve to be armed with the right tools to avoid medical errors and receive quality prenatal care.

It's hard, and I know it's not fair to have to put on your shoulders, especially with the worries you already carry with you about your health and your baby's health. But there is only one way to ensure you are not the victim of medical errors: Speak up when something feels wrong and demand action.

You've likely heard this message before. Still, I recognize that it is easier said than done. From the hundreds of women I have spoken with about this very topic, five very clear patterns emerge for why this is hard to put into action.

First, there is often literally no time in the appointment to have a lengthy discussion with your physician. Some patients feel so rushed that they can barely get their basic questions answered, let alone have a conversation about their worries about the baby. In many private conversations, medical professionals have shared their frustration with me as well about how little time they have with their patients. It's truly a lose-lose for everyone.

Second, many women confide in me that they are afraid of offending their doctors if they question the recommended treatment plan or raise concerns about their health that their doctor believes is not actually an issue. You want to be nice. You want to be polite. And you want to respect the relationship with the person who is taking care of your baby, but it comes at a cost of diminished communication with your care provider.

This leads to the third reason why it's frequently challenging for women to speak up about their concerns with their OB: They think their OB is the only expert in the room. Perhaps this has happened to you too. You recognize that you don't have an MD and therefore you doubt your instincts as well as how much you actually know about what you're going through. So even though your gut is telling you something's wrong with your OB's treatment recommendation, you stay silent—because who are you to challenge someone who spent decades of years receiving formal education and training in medicine when all you did was some Googling and talking to friends?

Fourth, women tell me they're tired of not being taken seriously and being waved off as just another anxious pregnant woman. They've tried speaking up, they've tried changing doctors but they're so tired of fighting for quality care that they become exhausted. That tiredness leads to acquiescence, a desire to stop fighting and just let things be. They tell themselves that their doctor probably has it covered and convince themselves that if there's a big issue, their OB will tell them. They feel disempowered and like they have no voice, so why does it matter if they speak up? This is a tremendous pitfall in our system that leaves patients wide open for medical errors.

Finally, the biggest one of all, and the one I work on with every single one of my clients no matter why they come to see me: They don't trust their bodies.

Psychiatrist Dr. Judith Orloff shares that our body is extremely powerful at communicating when something is wrong: "Intuition allows you to get the first warning signs when anything is off in your body that you can address it. If you have a gut feeling about your body—that something is toxic, weak or 'off'—listen to it."[5]

Trusting your body means understanding that there is not just a mind-body connection but a two-way mind-body *communication* that exists outside of our conscious awareness. Our brain is constantly sending and receiving messages about our internal organs, our bones, our nerves, even our cells, all without us realizing it's happening.

If there's a concern, our body tries to get our attention—at first, quietly. I call these "early warning whispers." But as we continue to ignore them, the message becomes louder and louder until we are forced to take action and get the help we need. Sometimes that's from our doctors, sometimes from other providers or treatment protocols. However, it always, *always*, starts with us listening to that little voice that never lies that says, "Pay attention. Something is wrong."

*

Fear had become our norm. It wasn't good. Not for me. Not for Sonil. Not for my pregnancy.

The sheer terror of waiting for the other shoe to drop, not knowing if it *would* drop, but knowing that if it *did*, it could have life-or-death consequences. That stress alone took a tremendous toll on both of us.

We were exhausted. Burned out. Fighting on fumes.

Sonil and I did our best to wade through it, leaning on friends and family to keep me entertained during the day and settling on the sofa for movies or TV shows together in the evening.

Just like every other week, one Thursday night Sonil and I finished an episode of *Once Upon a Time*. It was the perfect amount of fantasy and lack of reality that we needed to escape our day to day.

Something had felt different all week.

I couldn't quite pinpoint exactly what was different, but I knew something was off. I was still having contractions, but that wasn't new. They weren't any more painful—maybe slightly more frequent, but not enough to warrant a trip to the doctor sooner than my weekly cervical ultrasounds.

I slowly climbed up the stairs, with Sonil following behind me. This was his new thing in case I fell. Or . . . rolled. I'm not sure what he thought would happen now that my center of gravity was shifted. But it made him feel better, so I let it be. If walking behind me brought him a sense of comfort and peace, who was I to get in the way?

It was better than my latest source of comfort (reality TV).

I had started waddling, which made me giggle every time I walked. I was happy to be enjoying this milestone, one that comes so much earlier to vertically challenged women like me. I penguin-walked my way to the bathroom, getting ready for bed.

Not more than two minutes later, I stood at the door of the

bathroom, breathing fast and holding on to the door frame so I didn't fall down.

"What is it?"

He'd seen that face before. White as a sheet. Fear in my eyes. Silent. I'm never silent. From the moment I could talk, I haven't stopped.

There's a story my entire family knows of my uncle and aunt coming to visit us and wanting to take me to Burger King for lunch when I was 2. Before we left, my mom pulled me aside and told me to be polite and not talk to much.

"Come on. She's 2. Don't be so hard on her," my uncle told her.

Two hours later we came home, his hair disheveled and both of them exhausted as they handed me back to my parents. "I get why you said that now," he told her as he went to go lie down.

Words feed my soul. Talking is what I do best. So me, silent, means something big.

The words were stuck in my throat and took a couple of tries to get out. "I'm bleeding. I just had a huge bleed with a ton of clots."

Was it the subchorionic hematoma (the blood clot) back? Was it something else? I had no idea. But the new blood coupled with the fact that I felt something was wrong all week were enough to get my attention and want to do something about it—and fast.

The room was silent as he took in the magnitude of my words. The only sound we could hear was the dishwasher running in the kitchen. His mind raced with questions that he knew I didn't have the answers to.

"We have to call the on-call OB," I told him. "Can you grab the phone?"

I went to go lie down. Something was wrong.

I knew my OB wasn't on call that night, and I didn't want to have this conversation with a doctor who didn't know me and my history. There was no trust there like there was with my RE and my two MFMs.

I didn't have the energy to go through my entire complicated medical history on the phone. I left a message with the answering service and waited, Sonil holding my hand tight while I lay on the bed.

This man's eyes—the eyes I had fallen in love with on our first date— were filled with helplessness and sadness. He wanted to fix this for me, but he had no idea how. It broke my heart that this pregnancy, the one that was supposed to make us deliriously happy, had sucked the joy out of both of our hearts and filled it with heaviness, fear, and despair.

When the on-call OB called me back, I got her up to speed as fast as I could about my entire history.

IVF. OHSS. Hematoma. Dynamic cervix. Preterm contractions. So many problems. Weekly cervical ultrasounds. Bleeding tonight. Something's not right.

"There isn't a whole lot we can do for you right now. Take your progesterone suppository, rest tonight, and call your MFM in the morning to make an appointment."

That was the advice she had. That's it. Being in the periviable stage (after 20 weeks but before 24 weeks), doctors cannot do much for the baby to help it survive if it is born. So that was the answer I got.

We waited for 10 minutes.

My back was clenched. I was holding my legs tight, almost as if to prevent the baby from falling out. My head was spinning with so many thoughts.

She's the on-call OB. She doesn't really get my whole history even if she read about it.

But she said there's nothing we can do. Could going to the ER make it worse? Maybe being at home would be easier on my body.

Wait, though. What do you mean there's nothing they can do right now? How's that even possible?! *There* has *to be something I can do to help.*

What if something happens in the middle of the night? Could I wake Sonil up fast enough? There'd be no traffic to get to the hospital. But there's no traffic now.

Argh! Why don't MFMs give out their cell phone numbers? I'd really like to know what Dr. Kim has to say right now.

Stop! Stop driving yourself insane with this. Slow down.

Lizard brain. Grizzly bear. Run.

I hated how I was feeling. I needed to get a handle my anxiety and quickly. So, I started humming.

Deep breath in. Hum on the exhale. Deep breath in. Hum on the exhale.

The reverberations felt relaxing in my body. With every breath out, I sunk deeper into the bed, tension releasing from my legs, back, and shoulders. The thoughts faded against the sound of the humming.

When my mind finally became quiet and my body felt more relaxed, I was able to hear a little voice in the back of my head.

This voice was calm, cool, collected. It wasn't screaming and yelling at me, trying to get my attention.

It was quiet and direct. Like it always is.

What is your body telling you?

It was clear: Staying at home was the wrong move.

I yelled out to Sonil and he came sprinting into the room, his eyes wide with fear, thinking something scary had happened again.

Mental note: Stop yelling unless something horrible is actually happening. Poor guy is going to have a heart attack one of these days!

Whether you call it gut, instinct, intuition, inner light, your higher self—whatever it is for you—we all have this voice, but we so rarely listen to it because the bells and whistles that come with anxiety are so much louder.

When this voice speaks, like a newscaster giving the news, it's always calm. Cool. Collected. And direct. And it's always, *always* right.

You have to go to the hospital. Something's wrong.

Sonil scrambled to get everything together that we'd need for another trip to the ER. His backpack, jacket, and phone. A jacket for me and shoes that I could just slip on without having to bend down. Bending caused contractions.

"Grab your cell phone charger," I told him before we left.

I don't think we're coming home tonight. Something's wrong.

The drive to the hospital was unusually dark. I don't remember if it was because of my mental state or if there was actually no moon that night, but the darkness felt like it was descending on us.

"It's going to be like every other time," Sonil reassured both of us. "We're going to go and nothing will come of it and they'll send us home."

I was allowing his words to be an anchor for me to not completely drift away into my thoughts but I wasn't fully listening.

Something is wrong.

I directed Sonil to the labor and delivery after-hours door this time, instead of going to the ER. Thankfully my obsessively planning nature had given me the idea to watch the hospital's virtual tour a couple of weeks prior, so I knew exactly where to go.

He dropped me off and went to look for parking while I walked in, gingerly. The halls were quiet and empty. It felt eerie to be there so late at night when no one was around.

I followed the signs and, rounding a corner, I finally saw a handful of nurses huddled around a station. No one looked up or seemed especially happy to see me. Why would they? I didn't look very pregnant. In fact, in a big enough jacket, the only giveaway was my waddle. Maybe they thought I was lost.

When I spoke my voice cracked. I hadn't realized how terrified I was until I had to say the words out loud.

"I called the on-call OB a few minutes ago. I'm pregnant and I'm bleeding." *Did I just say that? Is this really happening?*

It all felt like a horrible nightmare that I couldn't wake up from.

One nurse grabbed a chart and told me to follow her to room 1. She got me settled, told me to change, and said the doctor would be by soon.

I got onto the bed just as Sonil walked in. I don't know if he was even breathing completely.

He had been scared most of this pregnancy, but this was the most scared I'd ever seen him. He just stood by me and held my hand. There was nothing to say.

The wait was short. The on-call OB and the same nurse came back in.

Just tell me this is all okay and I can go home.

The on-call OB was rattling on about how there was nothing they can do at this point in the pregnancy and how tomorrow it was very important that I see Dr. Kim. It was a scene out of Charlie Brown. I could hear her talking, I could hear her voice and see her mouth moving, but I couldn't really make out the words.

She checked me and it felt like the air was sucked out of the room. She went quiet, dropped her voice, and said, "You're 3 centimeters dilated."

I froze in shock. I couldn't make a sound. This is supposed to happen at the end of the pregnancy.

The end. Near the due date. 40 weeks.

I was only 22 weeks and 4 days. 22+4.

I was close to panicking. The alarms started in my head again, thinking of all the horrible things that could happen at any moment.

She tilted my bed in the Trendelenburg position (feet above my head so that gravity could help keep the baby in), got me started on a tocolytic (a medication to stop contractions), and started the paperwork to admit me to the hospital. I was clearly going nowhere.

My anxiety was all over the place, and I *knew* if I didn't get that under control, this baby could be born at any second. I could feel the tension in every part of my body. I needed to calm down. STAT.

I tried everything. Mantras. Visualizing. Deep breathing. Talking. Not talking. Nothing was working. I couldn't even get a handle on my breath. I couldn't find any anchors to help me calm down.

"Turn on some music," I told Sonil with urgency. "Turn it on now!"

He flustered a bit trying to find his laptop and connect to the Internet.

"What kind of music? Anything?"

"No!" Not just any kind of music.

I needed music that was soothing. That would calm my mind. That would release my body of tension. That would help me create a bubble—a cocoon—around myself and my little guy, so that no stress could get through.

There was no way I was going to let stress be the reason he was born that night.[6]

Soft rock had too many memories of teenage angst.

Pop songs reminded me too much of this pregnancy and all the drives to the ER when the radio was blaring to drown out our fears.

I didn't want to hear any songs that had come out earlier that year that remind me of our previous loss.

"Lata Mangeshkar. Play Lata Mangeshkar." A Bollywood legend. A singer from India who had been in the *Guinness Book of World Records* for recording the most songs in history.

She sang songs from my childhood, the days of predictability and joy. Songs that reminded me of my parents, unwaveringly strong and always there for me. Songs that would play in the background as we ran around the backyard or colored in the family room while my mom made homemade Indian food from scratch, every single night. Songs that played in the car as we dozed off to sleep after a day trips on the weekend.

This is what I wanted to hear. That peace, joy, blissful ignorance, and relaxation were what I needed to feel. Not just in my head, but more importantly in my body.

The melodies filled the room and I felt a cocoon being created around me. My body slowly started releasing tension, bit by tiny bit. Something was wrong. Something *big* was wrong. But this journey was not over. I wasn't ready.

I got 10 minutes of sleep that night.

The next morning, Dr. Kim and several nurses came in to check on me. They had been briefed and came as soon as they could to update me on the plan.

She pulled out several papers and discussed the horrible statistics about our possible future and the future of our son, should he miraculously survive, which was very unlikely if he was born any time in the next two weeks. She was trying so hard to walk the extremely fine line of telling us the harsh reality that lay ahead of us while trying not to crush our souls.[7]

Everything she was saying lit a fire in me.

She was telling me terrible statistics about my son's chance of survival or my chances of staying pregnant for 72 hours because she'd seen the worst. She's seen what happens most often.

But she hasn't seen me *go through this. How do we know those stats will apply to* me *and* my *situation?*

Ever since I was young, it had become a common saying in my family: "Don't ever tell Parijat she can't do something unless you want her to prove to you that she can."

"Parijat, you can't play table tennis. You're too small" would always result in me finding a paddle and inserting myself into a game, even when I could barely see over the top of the table.

"Parijat you can't run the race. Your asthma could flare up" meant I ran the race anyway, resulting in an asthma attack and my seventh-grade English teacher having to break into the girl's locker room so I could find my inhaler. "But I finished the race, didn't I?" I asked, between wheezes with a proud smile.

Just like that, I took it upon myself to prove Dr. Kim wrong.

When she left the room, I turned to Sonil. He looked like he'd been hit by a truck. We had heard some of the worst news in the entire pregnancy about our son's chance for survival, and I was terrified as well. But what kept coming to mind was one thought and one thought only: "She never said 100%."

Sonil fell into the chair that was by my bed, rubbed his face, and looked at me with total confusion.

"She never said 100% of babies in our situation don't survive. She never said 100% of babies will have neurological problems. She never said 100% of women at this stage of the pregnancy with these complications will deliver before viability. She never said 100%. If that's the case, there are babies who defy those odds. Who's to say we can't have one of those babies?"

He looked at me long and hard as hope and color returned to his face.

It sounds unbelievably optimistic, possibly giving you the impression that I'm a glass-half-full kind of person. I'm not. Seriously. In all my years as working in child and family therapy, doing research in clinical and developmental psychology, teaching clinical psychopathology, plus just being me, I had become a cynic and skeptic about most things related to health.

But something happens when your child's life is on the line. Something that pushes you into clarity and focus. It's like taking a pill from Bradley Cooper in *Limitless*, and all of a sudden you can understand things in a way that you wouldn't have been able to if the anxiety alarms were still ringing. Something that protects you and your body, helping you to turn off the deleterious stress response.

By listening to my inner voice, focusing on staying in my cocoon, and keeping my body tension free, I was able to focus on the only thing that mattered: helping myself stay pregnant. I was not going to allow any statistics, doctors, medications, or research to determine how long that was going to be.

When I deliver my son, whether that's two hours from now or two months from now, I want it to be because my body *knew it was time, because we had run out the clock on my pregnancy, squeezed every drop out of that sponge. Because it* actually was *time.*

This was not that time. There was more in me. I could feel it.

Calm. Cool. Collected. Direct.

Soon after, my OB, Dr. Edwards, came in. Her energy was much lower than Dr. Kim's, and it wasn't until she sat on my bed that I realized she had tears in her eyes.

"I'm so sorry," she said to me, holding my hand tight and looking at both of us.

She knew the statistics Dr. Kim had shared. She'd seen this play out too many times before, too. She knew the likelihood of my son's survival at this time, with everything else that had gone wrong up until this point, was close to zero.

"I'm going to be here a long time," I told her smiling and squeezing her hand back. "You'll see."

She smiled through her tears, nodding as you do to a child whose unwavering trust in Santa you don't want to crush. I knew she wanted to hope I was right but experience told her otherwise. She could see what lay ahead, the heart-shattering moments that no words can ever grasp, but she allowed me to have my hope. My delusions. Whatever she thought they were.

She had no idea how sure I was. This wasn't a delusion. This was my body telling me the truth.

The medical field, science, and technology that had all gotten us to this point had forgotten one critical aspect that impacts prognosis: the power of listening to and trusting my body.

She never said 100%.

This is not over yet. I know it. This fight is not over yet.

Calm. Cool. Collected. Direct.

❧

Anyone can learn to listen to their body and trust its messages at any time of their life. It doesn't require any special talent to do it and in fact has a tremendously positive impact for the prognosis of any health condition, even a high-risk pregnancy.

The first step in being able to listen to your body is to calm your anxiety and stop listening to the what ifs that are constantly circling in your head. You cannot hear your gut/instinct/little angel on your shoulder/inner light/intuition (whatever you call it) if you're feeling anxious. (Refer to Chapter 3 on how to manage anxiety.)

Anxiety is loud, like a siren ringing, trying to get your attention. But your gut, your intuition, your instinct is quiet. It doesn't flash bright red lights or scream at you when something is wrong. It speaks in a calm, cool, collected voice that tells you very directly, "Call the doctor" or "Go to the hospital" or "Something is wrong." But it will never yell, scream, or shout at you with sirens. The yelling you hear in your head is always anxiety.

It is physically impossible to hear the second voice when the first one is blaring. It's like trying to hear your cell phone ringing when the fire alarm is going off. When you're able to manage your anxiety, not only do you turn off the stress response, but you minimize the number of times the stress response will need to turn on because you will know how to trust your body instead of trusting the worries in your head.

Women who are going through a high-risk pregnancy most often feel stress and anxiety about the unknowns—namely, not knowing what to do if something bad happens. Do you go to labor and delivery or do you call your doctor? Do you page the on-call doctor or do you drink more water and see if it passes? It's scary thinking that every decision you make could have a tremendous impact on the health of your baby. It's overwhelming to feel that much pressure on your shoulders. However, this anxiety and the confusion that comes from that are immediately cleared up when you manage your anxiety so you can listen to that inner voice.

Whenever you notice the mind-chatter starting up again, like it did for me when I was lying on the bed at home trying to figure out what to do, take several long, deep breaths. The focus should be to physically relax your body into the chair or bed you're on. Turn off the stress response in your body and help your body activate your self-healing system.

Then ask yourself what your body needs in that moment. Get out of your head and into your body. I'll say it again: We can talk ourselves in and out of anything, but our body never lies.

When you're able to listen to your body, you build up a tremendous amount of confidence about your health, your treatment plan, and the next steps. That confidence inspires mental clarity and focus, which allow you to focus on the one thing that matters: your health and your baby's health.

When that's in clear focus, it becomes clear what you need to do and you no longer search for your doctor's approval to take that step. You will know when to go to the ER. You will know when something is wrong. You will also know when it's anxiety trying to trick you into thinking something bad is happening when it's not. When you experience it first-hand you can feel how simple it is to hear that voice—and how easy it is to trust it.

Every single one of my clients experiences a life-changing moment when they realize their body has been talking to them the whole time. It reinstates control when they were feeling helpless and it opens their eyes to realizing how much they can do for their bodies between appointments to help themselves stay pregnant.

One client in particular had a history of preterm delivery and started working with me when she developed preterm contractions at 25 weeks. By helping her lower her anxiety so she could listen to her body, she understood exactly which contractions were caused by her anxiety and which warranted a call to the doctor.

Toward the end of our work together, she shared a moment that she was most proud of during her pregnancy. She had gone in for a regular checkup that included a non-stress test (a noninvasive monitoring test for some women to track contractions and ensure baby is growing and developing well). Her contractions were strong at the beginning, as they always were because she was nervous about being at the doctor's office. As soon as the monitor picked up the contractions, the physician's assistant (PA) told her that she might need to go to the hospital and prepared her for an early admission.

My client recounted this moment with a smile of pride. She shared that she confidently turned to the PA and told her these contractions are not the ones that will land her in the hospital. She closed her eyes, and practiced some of the tools I'd taught her to activate her relaxation response, and, lo and behold, the contractions stopped. She laughed as she described the look of "utter shock" on the PA's face.

That confidence, that clarity, that unwavering belief in yourself to know what's happening in your body—that's what this is all about. The control and power that come from realizing that you have insight into and information about your body that no one else has and that you can do something to help yourself is mind-blowing. You know your body better than anyone, even your doctor, even if this is your first pregnancy. You can pick up those early warning whispers before any blood test, ultrasound, or physical exam.

I get goosebumps every time I see my clients experience it for themselves. It changes their life forever. That's not an exaggeration. Once you know how to turn down your anxiety to hear that little voice, that voice that never lies, doubt vanishes during pregnancy and even as you settle into motherhood and beyond. When it does try to rear its ugly head, you will also know how to trust your body over the worries in your head. Always.

Trust yourself and trust that your body is trying to help you stay pregnant. Your job is to speak up when you get these warning signals and to find someone who will listen to you and take you seriously. It's your doctor's job to figure out what's going on. Together, you'll figure out what to do about it—your doctor bringing their medical expertise to the table, you bringing your expertise on your body, both equally valuable and necessary to have a healthy pregnancy and baby.

As Mirka Knaster once said, "To connect with our bodies is to learn to trust ourselves, and from that comes power." The power to speak up. The power to fight for the best medical care. The power to release trauma, guilt, grief, and anxiety so you can be fully present for the little miracle you are growing right now. The power to manage your pregnancy complications, so your body can help keep you pregnant for as long as possible.

Get out of your head and into your body and release your body of tension. (See Appendix B for specific exercises.) Then ask yourself: *What does my body need right now?* Give it that. As the alarm bells silence and your mind becomes still, listen that quiet voice that's telling you what to do. Trust it. It will never steer you wrong.

Calm. Cool. Collected. Direct.

CHAPTER 7

Embracing Uncertainty

"If you surrender to the wind you can ride it."

—TONI MORRISON

Not knowing what's going to happen in the next hour, day, or week is one of the most challenging parts of a high-risk pregnancy. The most natural reaction to such uncertainty when so much is at stake—when *life* is at stake—is to plan. You plan for worst-case scenarios. You make contingency plans. You make backup plans for backup plans. Whether those plans are just in your head or written down, or you actually take action on them, the plans create some level of certainty, safety, and predictability.

They also create a false sense of relief and security.

While taking these preventative measures and preparing for the worst is smart and very practical, it doesn't alleviate the anxiety and worry you live with every day, wondering if you'll ever *have* to rely on these contingency plans. So, you double down on your efforts to make sure you don't need them.

You Google fervently to find stories of hope or information on how you can stay pregnant that your doctor may have forgotten to tell you. You analyze every symptom and try to understand where it's coming from. Was it a normal pain or was that a sign of something bad happening? You fight. All the time.

Who wouldn't? When your baby's life is on the line, what mother wouldn't fight with all her might all day, every day for as long as it takes?

That constant fight comes with a price.

Your physical and emotional stress is through the roof. You feel overwhelmed by each day, wondering how you're going to manage it all and stay sane.

Even worse is when it bleeds into your sleep, the "what ifs" getting louder as the house becomes quieter and darker. You might find it harder to fall back asleep too. Not only do you feel exhausted, but lack of sleep has been tied to many pregnancy complications such as preterm labor, premature rupture of membranes (water breaking too soon), and higher incidence of falling,[1] as well as placental abruption,[2] preeclampsia,[3] and preterm delivery,[4] so missing out on sleep is taking a physical toll on your body as well.

It might be scary to read all of this. I understand if you notice your heart racing a bit faster, your mouth feeling a bit dry, and starting to feel a bit jittery when you see how many factors play into the health of a pregnancy. I share this with you to also remind you that there is so much more in your control than you realize or are made to believe.

One way to achieve that is to give yourself permission to take a break from fighting all day, every day. You need it. Your body needs it. Even if you were being chased by a bear, you would find a place to hide and catch your breath, right? Similarly, during a high-risk pregnancy, you need to create that safe space where you feel comfortable stepping away from the fight for a few minutes or a few hours so your body can do what it does best when the self-repair system is on.

Your job is to give your body a chance to do just that. Where most women get stuck is not being able to turn off their brain. Many of them—and you may have done this, too—know they need to take a break. So they lie down. Put their feet up. Turn on the TV. Go sit by the pool. They try their very best to relax. But their mind just keeps going. They're making lists in their head. Going over test results in their mind. Making their way through the long line of "what ifs." Unfortunately, just because your body isn't moving doesn't turn off the stress response in your body.[5]

Tap into your "inner pharmacy" by activating your relaxation response, and *that* allows your body the opportunity to do what it does best. This self-repair mechanism needs a chance to be activated regularly to help you stay pregnant for as long as possible. To do this requires you to take a break from the fight and the way to do that is to surrender to your reality.

I don't mean surrender as in "wave the white flag and give up." There's a stark difference between surrendering and giving up. Giving up means you stop trying. You walk away from the fight, throw your hands up, and believe there is absolutely nothing you can do to help yourself or your baby.

Surrendering is about reframing your pregnancy complications or situation by accepting the reality. This includes accepting what's happening, what's in your control, and what is not.

Surrendering is about deeply understanding that your body is not against you. It's about fully believing and trusting that, despite the health challenges you and your baby are facing, your body's number-one goal is to help you and your baby be healthy and safe. Your job is to believe that with every cell of your body and to give your body the opportunity to heal itself to the best of its ability (sometimes with the help of medical interventions) no matter what complications you are experiencing.

Surrendering is also about checking the thoughts that float

in your head about yourself. Are you blaming yourself for these complications? Are you berating yourself for putting your baby's life in danger? Are you talking down to yourself for putting your career first and waiting so long to get pregnant? Are you telling yourself that you are not fit to be a mother, that you don't know what you're doing, that you are not good enough? Are you telling yourself you're worthy of help, support, and caring?

Most of my clients struggle with this. I did, too.

It's so easy to take the blame for your high-risk pregnancy and feel responsible for putting your baby and your family in this position and to feel like the only way through it is to fight. There's a very real fear women have that if they allow themselves to rest, that's when something bad will happen and they won't be prepared. In fact, resting and surrendering for a moment is exactly how you'll help yourself be prepared for whatever lies ahead.

🌱

"It's spa day!"

One of my favorite, most enthusiastic nurses sauntered into my room one morning. Every time she came in, I swear the room felt like more lights had been turned on.

It's like she was made of sunshine, and when she walked in, everything felt brighter.

I hadn't been able to get out of bed in 72 hours. That meant no bathroom, no shower, no clean hair. I felt gross. I bet I smelled gross, too.

She set up her iPhone on the shelf that housed my contractions monitor.

"Do you want me to turn the heartbeat monitor sound off?" she asked.

I had no idea turning off the sound was even an option. The decision felt ridiculously impossible though.

I fought so hard to get pregnant. Shouldn't I want to hear his heartbeat constantly? Shouldn't every part of him right now be so special that I want to be around it all the time? How would I feel if I lost him? Would I have wished I'd had more time with the sounds of life?

But I was exhausted. Even though I was in my cocoon, listening to my music and relaxing my body as much as I could, I could tell I wasn't totally relaxed. A part of my ear and brain were permanently fixed on the sound of that monitor, making sure I could still hear him—making sure nothing changed.

I thought I was fully in my cocoon, but with that monitor on, I could never truly be.

Am I a bad mom for wanting a break from the reassuring galloping sounds of my son's strong heartbeat?

Will I be okay if I don't hear them all the time or will I panic?

I didn't answer for what felt like minutes. I was judging myself so much I couldn't even make a decision. She could tell I was struggling with this yes-or-no question so she offered a solution:

"How about we turn it off for now? Get you into your spa day. And afterward if you want it on again, we can do that."

Before I could even ask, she added, "Don't worry. Even if we can't hear it in here, his heartbeat is still being picked up at the nurse's station. If anything happens, they'll come in and tell us."

I nodded in agreement, but I was still tense. I could feel it in my body. My back, my legs, my shoulders—everything was in a fighting stance (even though I was lying down) trying to keep my son inside.

Tears fell down the side of my face in embarrassment, that I, as a grown woman, had to be given a sponge bath. I didn't expect to be in this position until I was 95 (when hopefully it would be one of my children who would be caring for me).

I could feel the tension coming back as the shame creeped up.

Lizard brain. Grizzly bear. Run.

I took a few deep breaths and relaxed as best as I could into the uncomfortable bed in labor and delivery, a bed meant for short-term use, not meant for someone to lie in for multiple days without movement.

I can't believe this is happening.

These thoughts filled my head faster than the tub they were filling with water at the sink. *What happened to my life? To me?*

The nurse came back to my bedside and asked me to relax. She told me with a big smile that she was going to create a magical experience for me. I wiped my eyes and nodded, half wishing for it to be over so I could be alone.

She found a music station that played spa music, and the minute I heard the sound of chimes against the soft splash of water, I burst out laughing. She was taking this spa day very seriously.

It had been days, if not weeks, since the last time I had laughed— *really* laughed. It felt so good. Like a cold glass of water when you're parched.

Tension leaked out from my body and for the first time I felt relief. It felt like putting your head on the most luxurious pillow and allowing your body to melt into your bed after being on your feet for 18 hours straight. It was body- and soul-rejuvenating.

It was also a physical reminder to me that holding onto this physical tension is a choice. I could keep my muscles tense and believe that was helping me stay pregnant or I could rest and trust that, that will help me stay pregnant even more.

The relaxation felt like such a welcome gift that before my brain could catch up my body had already chosen. My eyes instinctively closed and I sunk into the bed.

Two more nurses had joined the spa day to help my nurse wash my hair and my body. The sound of them laughing, strategizing about how to wash hair my when I was lying upside down in bed, was a breath of fresh air.

More tension leaked out. That was what I needed, and in that moment I surrendered to them and let them take care of me.

I put my Type-A, control freak tendencies aside. I didn't have to figure anything out right then. I didn't have to be alert or focused. I didn't have to double-check that they were doing it right. I didn't have to make any decisions. I wasn't weak or incapable, flawed or broken for relaxing. I could choose to let this moment be about just this moment: getting much-needed rest and being taken care of while my body was still growing my baby.

So I lay there, felt my body melt into the lumpy bed, and surrendered.

*

It's mind-blowing how powerful your body is and what it's capable of even when you're in the middle of the biggest fight of your life. It takes my breath away every time I think of it and brings tears to my eyes every time I see it happen for my clients.

One woman I worked with had been in and out of the hospital since she hit 20 weeks. She already had a history of preterm delivery and this pregnancy had shown signs of pregnancy complications even earlier than her previous one. Her doctor had warned her that she may deliver even earlier than her first and she should prepare herself for not making it too far into the third trimester.

After her third stint in the hospital, during which she described yelling at her partner and her mother-in-law purely out of stress, she reached out for help. She was fiercely determined to stay pregnant longer than her doctor was predicting and wanted to know what more she could do. Our work together, as with all of my clients, was about allowing her body to heal and recover from the physical and emotional stress she was under. Not only did she never return to the hospital for an overnight visit, her preterm contractions became more infrequent, and when they did arise, she knew exactly how to stop them at home. Her blood pressure decreased and she developed such a confidence in her body that she would reassure her nurses not to worry because she knew what her body was capable of.

When you can tap into this "built-in pharmacy," you can fully experience how many tools we have at our disposal to help ourselves stay pregnant. Surrendering to your reality gives you a much-needed reprieve from the fight, which can tremendously improve your health during pregnancy. It's all about allowing your body to do what it is trying to do and what it does best: help you recover and heal from the impact of stress so you can stay pregnant.

Practicing mindfulness is one powerful tool to help you do just that and can be powerfully effective especially during pregnancy.[6] I'll admit, this is a bit of a New Age buzzword right now, but it really does work. Mindfulness is "the practice of cultivating nonjudgmental awareness in day-to-day life."[7] But let's be honest, it's a huge concept that can feel overwhelming to take on when you have so much already weighing on you during your high-risk pregnancy.

My take on mindfulness, and how I teach it to my clients, is to get out of your head and into your body. Whether you're sitting at your desk at work, lying on the couch in the evening, or stuck in a hospital bed, your mind is likely swirling with thoughts that are strong, are powerful, and feel believable. Stopping those thoughts is important but the task can feel like trying to plug up a burst dam with a wine bottle cork.

My best advice: forget your thoughts and focus on your body.

This can be really challenging for most people. Almost every one of my clients finds this extremely powerful when they are able to do it, but at the beginning find it difficult. It's not their fault, nor yours. Most of us grow up very disconnected from our bodies. We get so caught up in our thoughts, trusting them as the ultimate truth, and handing over our bodies to medical professionals, medications, or alternative providers to fix when there's a problem. We look to a thermometer to tell us if we have a fever or a scale to tell us if we've gained or lost enough weight, when our bodies are sharing this information with us all the time. This is one of the biggest reasons we miss the early warning signs that we discussed in the previous chapter.

Learning to listen to your body and be present in your body not only helps you through a health crisis like a high-risk pregnancy but is a life-long skill that will serve you in any situation that you find yourself going forward.

The easiest way to practice mindfulness by getting into your body is to put your hand on an object that is nearest to you. Maybe it's a pillow, a throw blanket, a water bottle, or even this book. Close your eyes and feel that object, describing it with as many words as you can. Try doing it for 30 seconds As this becomes easier, try for 60 seconds or longer.

A more advanced version of this exercise is to focus more deeply in your body and notice bodily sensations.

Do you have pain? Where is it? Describe it. Do you feel muscle tension? Where? How does it feel? Do you feel achy? Name the spots.

Focus also on positive sensations too. What parts of your body feel relaxed or comfortable? Or if you're having a particularly difficult day, which parts feel the least bad?

Describe them. Focus on them. Put your energy and your attention on the parts of your body that feel good to you in the moment. If you can experience a positive sensation physically once, you can create that sensation again. (For a more information about this exercise, see Appendix A.)

Here's an example of what I mean.

I worked with a woman who had a history of miscarriages and PPROM (her water broke very early in pregnancy). When she came to me, her biggest complaint—aside from her fear of losing another baby of course—was hip pain. We worked on these mindfulness exercises together, helping her get into her body and be present with it beyond the pain. It was very challenging for her; the pain was excruciating and she had trouble seeing and feeling past it. One day, she visited a relative and took a bath in their tub, and her pain dissipated. She felt her body relax and she described it as feeling like she could breathe again.

I asked her to spend time describing that physical sensation to herself, to use as many words as she could to help this sensation become a body memory, one that her hips could recall at any time. Then, we used those words to help guide the tools she would use to help re-create that sensation in her hips even when she wasn't in the bath.

What this did for her, and what it will do for you, is help you become fully attuned to your body so you know how to move it, how to treat it and what to give it to re-create the positive sensations you're experiencing. Those positive sensations, such as being pain-free in the hip and feeling relaxed in the shoulders, have a ripple effect both physically and emotionally.

Physically, when you can experience pain-relief or relaxed muscle tension, the stress response shuts off, which improves inflammation, pain, and muscle tightness (including preterm contractions), lowers blood pressure, and helps create a positive feedback loop physically.

Emotionally, it brings back a sense of control because you can actually feel your body changing as you re-create that experience. It aids in creating a new narrative about your story, from one in which you're a victim to your complications and health problems to one where you're in charge of how you feel physically despite the diagnosis. This shift can alleviate your mood by reducing feelings of helplessness and can calm your anxiety, which is also essential to quieting the stress response and triggering the relaxation response that's built into your body.

Best of all, it gets you out of the "what ifs," out of obsessing about the future, and out of the contingency plans. It brings you to the moment at hand and forces you to be present right here, right now. That is what mindfulness is all about.

🍂

When I was in high-school, I ran cross-country. I loved the long runs. Feeling my legs carry me for 10 or 12 miles. My arms pumping energy through my body. The quiet. The stillness as I got into a groove and kept running, with no end in sight. It felt meditative and soul-cleansing for a couple of hours with no distractions.

Cross-country was exactly what my Type-A personality needed. Because the runs were so long, I couldn't think about the end. The finish line, where I ended up, how I got there, what it would feel like, how to strategically time and plan the end of the race—those weren't on my radar for most of the run. It forced me to pace myself and go slow.

My entire focus was on where I was and how to get to the next mile marker, sometimes the next half-mile if the run was particularly difficult. But that's it; that's all there was.

My mind was empty as I allowed my body to carry me forward in the way it instinctively knows how to do. I surrendered to the journey, trusting that the finish line would come and believing that my body could carry me there.

Cross-country was such a powerful practice of mindfulness, something I hadn't realized until I was in the hospital with my high-risk pregnancy.

A high-risk pregnancy isn't a sprint, even though I treated it as such until my hospital days. It's a marathon, and I was in it for the long game.

My body had stopped, obviously. I was on bed rest for months at home. I wasn't exercising or going to work. But my mind hadn't stopped at all. In fact, in response to how little I was doing physically, I was trying to make up for it mentally, by creating contingency plans, researching, and thinking about what could go wrong.

Truthfully, though, practicing mindfulness was extremely challenging for me. Staying focused on the present was almost impossible some days because I just wanted to know that we'd be okay. *Just tell me we'll survive this.*

The problem was that I was feeding into the problem.

The hamster wheel that doesn't stop was keeping the stress response on in my body.[8]

Lizard brain. Grizzly bear. Run.

I was convinced I didn't have a choice about that until the choice became: *deliver now and lose the baby* or *do whatever you can to buy a few more hours or a few more days and give him a chance.*

🌿

The choice is yours, too. You *can* take charge of your pregnancy by surrendering to your reality by practicing mindfulness and giving your body the rest it needs to help you stay pregnant. If you're reading this and thinking about previous losses or previous preterm deliveries and blaming yourself for that happening, stop.

It's not your fault. You didn't cause whatever happened in your past. It wasn't because of something you did or you didn't do.

You're here now because you want something different this time around. Choosing to calm your stress response and surrender to your reality so your body can focus on self-repair, even if everything is falling apart around you, is exactly what you can do—what you *need* to do.

Now is a good time to stop and ask yourself: *Am I ready to surrender? Am I ready to allow my body the rest and recovery that it needs to help me stay pregnant for as long as possible?*

🌿

I closed my eyes. The nurse added some soap to her washcloth and the waft of lavender came over me.

Home.

It reminded me of home. Of comfort. Of security and safety.

I allowed my nurse to massage my scalp without feeling guilty about the self-care. I gave myself to the gentle sounds of spa music, bringing a sense of quiet and calm to a sterile, chaotic environment.

I surrendered to the moment and, for a while, I forgot where I was and why I was there.

When she moved the two monitors that I'd been attached to for days, I felt a release from my belly. Like when you loosen your belt after a huge holiday meal. Ahhh, so good.

The monitors were a physical reminder of the tenuous situation we were in. Even if my mind wasn't focused on them, my body was paying attention and not able to fully relax until that moment for the few seconds they were off.

Because the monitors took up most of my tiny, 23-week belly, and because I was lying with my feet above my head, I hadn't really felt him move since I landed in the hospital. He was so tiny that feeling movements was still inconsistent. With gravity working toward my head, he also lay higher up in my belly where I couldn't feel him as easily even when he did kick and punch.

"Can you wait to put the monitors back on for a second?" I asked, breaking the silence.

She held them in her hands as I put my hand on my belly for the first time in three days and said hi. I talked to him like I used to at home and, as if he knew something had changed, he suddenly became active, head-butting me and kicking me where my hands were.

I cried and laughed as he so clearly responded to my voice, and he knew the difference between the monitors and my hands. It was a humanizing moment during a time when I had started to feel like nothing more than an incubator. I let myself feel that connection and that joy that I had been so scared to feel since I had landed in the hospital and thought I would lose him.

I was still terrified he would not survive but I was so grateful to have made that particular memory, which I have not forgotten to this day.

When Sonil came back into the room, even he could feel the change in the air. There was a sense of levity and, as relaxed as I felt in my body, he could see it on my face. I could see his whole body relax, too. The relief was palpable for everyone.

*

We don't know what's going to happen tomorrow or five minutes from now. The phrase *anything is possible* really does mean anything. Things could take a turn for the worse as you fear, but they could also take a turn for the better because you're giving your body the opportunity to rest, relax, and recover from the stress.

Give yourself permission to surrender to the uncertainty. As much as I know you would do anything for a crystal ball to tell you what to expect, uncertainty is your reality right now. Allow yourself to release the tension from the unknowns, put away the plans, and be fully present in this very moment by being in your body. Give yourself relief from your stress. You have the power to set the stage for your own miracle story by surrendering from the fight and giving your body a chance to rest and recover so you're prepared for whatever lies ahead.

CHAPTER 8

Healing with Hope

"Where there is hope, there is life."

—Dr. Jerome Groopman, MD

In the face of a health crisis, certain pieces of advice start to sound like a broken record.

Think positive.

Look on the bright side.

Everything will be okay.

You've likely heard many such encouragements from loved ones who mean well and are hoping for the best for you and your family. Maybe you've even told yourself some of these pieces of advice yourself, especially when you find yourself feeling down, negative, or hopeless. You know you shouldn't, or don't want to feel that way, but you can't seem to shake it.

Yes, optimism and hope for the future are essential for health. Decades of research have shown the connection between pessimism and increased risk of cardiovascular disease, lowered immunity, and increased inflammation, while optimism has shown the exact opposite: protection against heart disease, improved immunity, and a reduction of inflammation.[1] Hope has a similar effect on your immune system as optimism.[2]

However, thinking positively and being optimistic are easier said than done for most women during a high-risk pregnancy. With the consistent barrage of bad news, the anxiety from uncertainty, and new diagnoses popping up like moles you want to whack away, the emotional experience of a high-risk pregnancy can be tumultuous. You might feel like you're on a roller-coaster, being jerked around from one side to the other, wondering if your harness is on tight enough to keep you safe.

You might be trying everything you can think of to stay hopeful—focusing on the positives, making gratitude lists, telling yourself that everything is fine—but it may not be working nearly as well as you had thought it would. You aren't alone.

Countless women who contact me lament that their efforts of positive affirmations and mantras haven't helped them with their anxiety or low mood. I'm not surprised, to be honest. Affirmations and positive self-talk have been shown to be ineffective in people who are already experiencing anxiety or low mood because using them has shown to minimizes the real emotional experience you're having, adding pressure, guilt, and blame for not feeling as happy or as hopeful as you think you should.[3]

I once worked with a client who told me she was frustrated because she was grateful for being pregnant after fertility treatment and a miscarriage as well as for having crossed a major pregnancy milestone. But she still felt so down. She felt helpless. She felt scared and anxious all the time. Once she got the official diagnosis of a pregnancy complication, she broke down and didn't know what to do. All the negative thoughts came rushing back, her fears about losing the baby took over, and she felt helpless to protect her baby.

That's when she reached out, because she thought I would teach her to be more positive.

I didn't, because it doesn't work.

We can think ourselves in and out of anything. Thoughts are fleeting, even though they feel like facts. They're unreliable, subjective, and based entirely on context like your mood, how well you've slept, how hungry you are, and so forth. So we never worked on changing her thoughts, and I recommend you don't spend time trying to change your thoughts either. Instead, I want to show you, as I showed her, how to develop a sense of fortitude, determination, and resilience in her pregnancy that naturally flows into positive thinking, more hope, and more optimism that lasts no matter what lies ahead.

🌿

The day after my spa day, after a reassuring conversation with Dr. Edwards and Dr. Kim, the decision was made to move me to the mother-baby unit. There was no antepartum unit at the time, so I was given a room in the area with all the women with their babies.

The nurses did a good job of putting me in a room as far away from the commotion of crying newborns as possible, but it was clear to me what the room was for. It was one of the smaller rooms in the unit. It was so small there was hardly any space for a baby bassinet.

"Oh, how nice. They have a room that's the perfect size for you!" Sonil said.

It's not for me. It's for the women who don't have babies rooming in. For the women whose babies are not with them. Who are in the NICU. Who don't make it.

That was the reality. I needed a room like that, and I hoped that all of the flowers, balloons, and gifts that we'd received would rid the room of that dreaded feel and brighten it up.

Something about being in that room didn't feel right to me, though.

I was feeling anxious, and the monitors showed it with plenty of spikes for the contractions. The mother-baby nurse wasn't familiar with constant monitoring. Obviously. Her patients aren't pregnant anymore. That made me really nervous and distrustful.

Lizard brain. Grizzly bear. Run.

My team of babysitters created shifts for themselves. My parents and best friend took turns sitting with me, playing games with me to pass the time, and helping me keep my mind off of what was going on while Sonil was at work.

"This is good!" my dad told me as we prepared to move what amassed to an entire cart full of belongings to my new room. He, Sonil, and my mom were hopeful that if I stabilized in the mother-baby unit, maybe I could go home.

The pit in my stomach told me otherwise.

I needed less anxiety. I needed less tension in my body. I wanted music. I wanted security, and it didn't feel like mother-baby was the place to be. But I didn't push back. Not speaking up here was one of only two regrets I have in my entire pregnancy.

I needed things to turn around. I was desperate for some good news. And I was exhausted. So instead of listening to my body, which was telling me something I didn't want to hear, I tuned it out and went along with the plan.

That afternoon, one of the OBs in Dr. Edwards's group practice came in. He was an older man with a sense of calmness and sturdiness about him. His voice was very deep, and he moved with an air of certainty and confidence. He reminded me of George Clooney from his *ER* days.

He had no answers for me—nothing new to tell me about what to expect or what could happen. We'd gone through the conversations with Dr. Kim and Dr. Edwards as well as a neonatologist multiple times.

He sat next to my bed, his long legs barely fitting between the chair and my guardrail.

He told me his daughter-in-law was due about the same time as I was. He took off his glasses, rubbed his eyes, and looked directly into mine.

"I'm really pulling for you," he said to me. "We all are."

Those words meant more than I could ever say to him, and I'm not sure I ever fully thanked him for sharing that. I couldn't quite find my anchors to ground me from my anxiety but it felt like he had wrapped me in a thick, fuzzy blanket, shielding me from the harsh cold.

I had a great team, and the team was growing by the day. From nurses and doctors in the practice rooting for me (and later I found out advocating for me against hospital bureaucracy) to friends and family from around the world visiting, sending flowers and care packages, and asking for prayers on our behalf.

I felt the love from every corner of the universe being sent our way. I needed it to combat the uneasiness I felt being in that room.

The next day, the mother-baby nurse came back and asked me to try using a bedside toilet. They wanted to take the catheter out. Fear of infection. And they wanted me to get out of bed and get moving a little if I could.

It felt wrong. I told her. I pushed back. I was insistent that this was a bad idea. But that was the order: get me up to just use the bathroom, and then I could lie in trendelenburg the rest of the time.

Something felt wrong the minute I stood up. Something felt very wrong when I sat on that makeshift dark gray, plastic bedside toilet.

Something felt very, very wrong when I went back to bed. I didn't know what.

No one wanted to check me to see what was going on. She just asked me to stay calm, breathe, drink water, and relax.

Lizard brain.

This was more than needing to relax. This was more than dehydration. Something was wrong.

I was sweating. I was breathing fast as the neonatologist came in to talk to me again about new statistics now that I was 23 weeks along. What was my son's chance of survival now? What was his chance of long-term physical, mental, neurological disability now?

The numbers were still awful and scary. Odds were still very much stacked against us.

Grizzly bear.

I heard him talking. My best friend was sitting beside me, my mom in a chair by my feet, listening and taking it all in. I could see his mouth moving. I was getting bits and pieces. But I wasn't fully there.

Something was wrong.

I bit my knuckles. I started breathing even faster.

Run.

As he finished talking to us, I felt a bit of relief—physically and emotionally. My body sunk into the bed. My breathing slowed. It felt like I had been in a vicious battle that had finally ended so I could rest.

"The news is better!" my best friend said cheerfully trying elevate the mood in the room after the neonatologist left. She turned to look at me to gauge my reaction of the recent conversation.

I didn't respond. I closed my eyes. I was exhausted. I needed calm. I couldn't think. I could barely move.

I breathed.

In. Out. In. Out. In.

The bed carried all of my weight. I had no energy left to hold myself up.

A few seconds later, my eyes shot open and met hers.

In a voice barely above a whisper I said, "I think my water broke."

She gasped. "I'm calling the nurse!" she said, scrambling to press the call button numerous times to get someone's attention.

My mom ran out of the room to call Sonil to tell him to rush to the hospital.

I lay frozen.

The mother-baby nurse flew into the room followed by a new labor and delivery nurse—I'll call her Valeria—who took immediate charge. She ripped off the blankets I was under and using pH strips checked the fluid on the bed.

"It's amniotic fluid," she said confidently and loudly. This was meant to trigger a chain of reactions to rush me back to labor and delivery. Because my water had broken. At 23+2.

"Is this your first?" she asked with kind eyes as her hands moved quickly to prepare me for the ride down to L&D.

"No, my second. We lost the first," I croaked out. Sadness sat on my chest like an elephant but I couldn't breathe enough to actually cry.

There was nothing but a tornado of panic in my head and a whirlwind around me of nurses pulling up guardrails, grabbing my belongings, and rushing me.

They were going fast. Speed- walking.

I could feel the rush of the air on my face as I lay there, on my back, eyes fixated on the tiles on the ceiling.

How could I have been so wrong? This can't be happening. How could I have been so wrong?

Since my diagnosis of dynamic cervix and preterm contractions about five weeks prior, I had had a vision of bringing this baby home. I don't remember if it came to me in a dream at night or a dream during a nap or when I was half-asleep in front of the TV at home.

I could see us, so clearly, as if it were a memory. Sonil in front, wearing his favorite tan sweater and jeans, holding a gray infant car seat in his hands. Me following behind in a black shirt and gray pants. Both of us climbing the stairs from the garage to the living room. Happy. Ecstatic. On the other side. With our little boy at home.

During every ultrasound and after every appointment with Dr. Kim, I thought of that image and felt safe. With every contraction at home, I remembered that image and felt confident. It calmed my body and my mind.

That was a vision, an image, I'd held on to for weeks as security and comfort. It felt so real. It wasn't just in my head; I could feel it in my bones that he was coming home even though medically all signs pointed otherwise.

I just knew it, though. I knew it more clearly and more assuredly than I knew my own name.

And yet there I was, being rushed back to labor and delivery. Back to Room 1, this time in a state of emergency because I still hadn't hit viability. Just 10 minutes prior the neonatologist told us about the horrible statistics that could become my son's life—if he survived. We were going to lose him.

How could I have been so wrong?

The room looked completely different. It was dark except for some very bright spotlights. It felt like there were about 176 people in the room. It was loud. People talking, bustling, moving around.

I had just spent a little more than four days in this room and yet it looked completely unfamiliar—not my safe haven, as it felt before.

They lined up the mother-baby bed right next to the L&D bed and a nurse asked me to move over.

"Come on! You can do it. Scooch over!" the nurse motioned to me from the other side.

No. I couldn't do it. I didn't want to move.

Moving meant I had to accept the reality that my water broke. Moving meant I was accepting that after all of this, I was going to lose my baby. Moving meant this was over.

I was not ready to stop fighting. I was not ready for this to be over. I wasn't ready to move.

So I lay frozen. Completely motionless. There was so much commotion and movement around me, but not a cell in my body moved. I felt paralyzed.

Valeria reached out and gave me her hand. She looked straight into my eyes and said, "Hold on to me. I've got you. You can do this."

She was strong. Physically but also emotionally. She was exactly the rock I needed: unwavering, confident, direct.

I grabbed her hand, held it tight as she squeezed my hand back, and with her guidance and the help of several other nurses glided on to the labor and delivery bed.

The lights were blinding and I could hardly see what was happening.

Before I knew it a neonatologist, one I hadn't yet met, was standing next to me, cozy in her black fleece, hands in her pockets.

If he's born right now, do you want to resuscitate?

I knew we'd be asked this question. Our entire medical team had prepared us for this question. It wasn't an option a few days before, but the hospital policy was that after 23 weeks it was the parents' decision. They often advised against it, but it was our choice.

Thoughts still hadn't returned to my head and instead I was starting to lose feeling in my hands and feet. Without even realizing it, I was opening and closing my hands to get some feeling back.

"Are your hands tingling?" Valeria asked.

I nodded.

"You're hyperventilating." She showed me how to breath into my cupped hands over my nose and mouth until I could slow down my breath.

Remember that cocoon? It was *long* gone. This girl who was *so* good about recognizing when anxiety was affecting her pregnancy—the girl who didn't consider being anxious as part of her identity—was now hyperventilating.

Who had I become? Was this actually happening? I was going to lose this baby who I had been so sure would come home with us. How could I have been so wrong?

I had a flash thought of what it would be like to experience labor and delivery only to have this baby lose his life in my arms. I thought of a good friend who had experienced just that about a year prior. I couldn't do it.

I'm not strong enough to do this.

As if Valeria could read my mind, she said, "Take pictures."

Had I just shared my fears out loud? I was 90% sure I was just thinking them, but maybe I had spoken out loud?

"Most couples don't want to hold the baby or take pictures, but take the pictures," Valeria said. "I promise you'll want them later."

I couldn't even wrap my head around this. *This is not happening. This cannot be happening.*

I wanted to rewind.

Was there anything I could do to go back just 15 minutes, back to when he was safely inside this bubble in my belly. Please? Anything?

Sonil came flying into the room. Someone had briefed him on what had happened. He sat next to my bed and held my hand tight as the neonatologist repeated her question.

"If he comes right now, do you want to resuscitate?"

He looked into my eyes with a fierceness and a fear I'd never seen.

I had started breathing again and slowly the feeling in my hands and legs returned, as did clarity of thought.

Another one of my perinatologists, Dr. Weyland, had come in. I was 5–6 cm dilated, and based on how early it was in the pregnancy, I didn't need more than 1–2 cm more until it would be enough to deliver my son. (You don't need a full 10 cm to deliver a baby in the second trimester.)

We didn't need to have a conversation in that moment. We'd been talking for days about how we would handle it if we had to answer this question about resuscitating our child.

I looked at the neonatologist and told her *yes,* we wanted to resuscitate.

Is that the right choice for everyone? Nope. Are couples bad parents for choosing not to? Nope. This was our decision about our child given our situation—nothing more.

With that, the neonatologist left to prepare in case I delivered, because it could have happened at any moment.

Dr. Weyland gave me a choice. I could start on magnesium sulfate, an IV medication and the strongest medication we have access to stop preterm contractions, or I could let nature take its course.

Sonil was still holding on to me tight. "I will support you no matter what you want to do."

Through tears I told him, "This whole time my body has had so much trouble. There have been so many problems but it's been with me. Not with him. We have to give him a chance."

He nodded and I told Dr. Weyland to bring on the magnesium. I wasn't hyperventilating anymore but my anxiety was all over the place.

As the nurses filed out of the room, Valeria went to get the IV ready.

"I've had patients who have gone on to stay pregnant for weeks or months after their water broke," Dr. Weyland said.

Insert sound of screeching car brakes.

Wait—*what?!* I had no idea that was even remotely possible.

Suddenly it felt like the room was filled with air and I took my first real breath all afternoon.

She described to us several cases of her patients who had gone on to deliver near term or at term even after their water had broken. Does it happen for everyone? No. But the fact that it could happen to some meant it *could* happen for me.

Tears filled my eyes. Sonil and I both started breathing. We held onto each other's hands so tightly our knuckles were white.

Dr. Weyland left us. The room had come to a complete halt. It was quiet again, only me and Sonil and this little bean that was still in me. Maybe for a few hours. Maybe for a few days. Hopefully for a few weeks or more.

No one knew. But what we did know is that there was a chance for a miracle.

Hope. It was back with a force like never before in this pregnancy.

It meant breath. It meant life. It meant everything.

"We're not meeting him today," I told Sonil, my voice finally losing its shakiness and gaining some strength. "Today is not the day."

Calm. Cool. Collected. Direct.

Valeria came back and gave us the rundown of what to expect on magnesium. In a nutshell, it makes women feel absolutely horrid.

She warned me one of the most common symptoms is feeling like your face is on fire and she set up a fan to turn on as soon as that happened. She hooked up a port in my arm, hung the bag, and started the bolus (a highly concentrated short dose that would be followed by a much lower long dose).

I closed my eyes and settled into my tilted bed, with the blood rushing to my head. My feet felt like they were soaring above me.

I vowed to never go on an upside down roller coaster again.

I closed my eyes and took a deep breath, and Valeria turned on the IV. Within a few minutes I could feel it.

My head felt like it was being crushed by a big rig. My face, just as Valeria had predicted, felt like someone had lit it on fire.

A throbbing headache pulsated between my temples. My eyeballs felt warm, and my eyelids felt like they were made of cement.

I wanted to ask for a head massage. And some extra blankets. For all the heat that was in my face, I felt the rest of my body had turned into an icicle.

The room was so quiet. When did everyone leave? Was Valeria still in the room? Where was my family?

I slowly opened my heavy eyelids to see my entire family standing by my bedside.

Parents and brother on one side, best friend and husband on the other. I knew they'd be worried but I wasn't expecting this.

They were staring down at me, their faces unmoving.

Morose.

Tear-stained.

Devastated.

They looked at me like I had just died.

"You guys are creeping me out. Can you please stop staring at me and go sit down?"

For a couple of seconds they didn't know what to say, and then all of them burst into a roar of laughter—laughter of relief, release, and so much gratitude that we were on the other side of this awful scare.

Valeria ushered them all to seats and helped them get comfortable.

"She's back," my dad said with tears in his eyes.

Sounds filled the room again, this time of jokes and light-hearted stories from my childhood.

"Do you guys remember the time she was 3 and picked up the phone and called some man in Japan?" my mom started. Everyone jumped in, piling on memories of times I'd done something that was so *me* that made them all laugh.

These were the sounds of comfort. The sounds of home. The fuel that I needed to fill my mind and body of hope and rebuild the strength to keep fighting.

Warm tears fell from my eyes down the side of my face. Today was not the day I was going to meet my son. The anxiety was gone and I could feel it in my body. Today was not the day.

Calm. Cool. Collected. Direct.

*

When you hear bad news during your high-risk pregnancy, whether it's bloodwork with concerning results, an ultrasound that shows growth issues for the baby, or your doctor's admittance of uncertainty about what is going to happen next, it's natural to go into shock. Your mind might go blank. You might cry. Maybe you might even hyperventilate, like I did.

All of that is a very normal reaction to bad news, especially news that carries life-threatening consequences for you and your baby. What happens next helps you set the foundation for optimism and hope.

Some women react by feeling crushed by the news, feeling like they're falling into the hole of helplessness. They might feel like everything's over, there's nothing more they can do, that they have failed their baby.

Other women stay in denial, convinced that if they just think positive and hope for the best everything will work out and they'll feel better. They suppress their emotions thinking it will help move passed the fear and anxiety.

Both of these reactions, though common, trigger the stress response in your body, which has a cascading effect on the health of your pregnancy, from increased inflammation to lowered immunity, elevated blood pressure, or blood glucose reading to an increase in preterm contractions.

If you've found yourself following either of these paths, it's okay. We've all done it. When we are overwhelmed and scared, it's easy to go into survival mode or to feel crushed by our reality. I hyperventilated! I get it. It really is okay. It's not the end of the world, because you can learn a new way to cope.

The next time some bad news comes your way, allow yourself to have your initial reaction of shock, sadness, anger, denial—whatever it is. Then, when you feel ready, ask yourself one question: *What can I do to help myself beat the odds?* In other words, ask yourself what you can do to improve your chances of a positive outcome for this moment.

It's an extremely powerful question because it puts you in the driver's seat of your situation. When you ask yourself what you can do, you're opening your mind up to consider in- and out-of-the-box solutions that can help you. By asking yourself how you can beat the odds, you're acknowledging for yourself the possibility that you can experience a miracle too.

Research has suggested that patients who respond with such a fierce determination to overcome the odds have a much better prognosis for health conditions like cancer and heart disease than patients who believe the "doom and gloom" that's often set forth by their doctors.[4]

In fact, taking an active role in your health by asking this question has been shown to lower the stress response,[5] which in turn ignites the self-repair mechanism, which is essential to helping manage existing complications and lower your risk of developing new ones.

Several months ago, I worked with a woman who was on hospital bed rest and feeling terrified of losing her baby. She was just at the beginning of the third trimester, her water had broken, and she was scared about what lay ahead. She reached out to me mostly because I had been on hospital bed rest, had experienced PPROM (her water broke preterm), and also had delivered prematurely. She wanted to get some insider information on what to expect. She was not expecting our first conversation to revolve around her asking herself what she could do to beat the odds.

She was convinced there were no odds to beat and there was nothing she could do to change them. Finding an answer was challenging for her because of this, so I asked her to repeat the question over and over to herself until something came to her. I reassured her we weren't looking for a cure or a magic solution. Asking this question was meant to bring her to the other side of despair: the land of hope and optimism.

She repeated the question several times and then I witnessed her entire demeanor change. Her face brightened, her shoulders dropped, her chest rose with a deep breath. And she smiled a small smile.

I asked her what came to her and she said, "Nothing yet"—but just asking this question made her feel powerful, something she had not felt in the several days since being admitted to the hospital. I could see hope returning. I could see her feeling more optimistic about her outlook. We discussed the realities of her situation and the likelihood of her delivering preterm still, but we spent far more time brainstorming how she could help her body help her stay pregnant.

We worked together to master several techniques that elicit the relaxation response. (See Appendix B for a list of recommended tools to try.) By doing them, she was able to manage her preterm contractions (as could be seen by a change on the monitors), which helped her feel even more in control, improved her mood, and helped her stay hopeful because she could feel immediate changes in her body that *she* was creating.

This is not about denying the reality or believing that your doctor is overstating how bad the situation is. It's about acknowledging the really challenging position you're in, that the odds are stacked against you, but also finding things you can do to help yourself overcome those odds. It's, of course, not a guarantee of any particular outcome, but it is a guarantee that when you search for ways to help your body stay pregnant, no matter what happens, you'll know you did everything you could to help your baby stay inside for as long as possible. You won't look back on your pregnancy with regrets, wondering "what if?"

❦

The next evening, Dr. Kim came to see me.

"Fifty percent of women deliver within 24 hours after their water breaks," she told us. We had already crossed 26 hours. "Another 25% deliver within seven days."

This data rocked Sonil's core. This was the exact opposite of the hopeful message we'd heard just one day prior from Dr. Weyland. The look on his face was of utter devastation. A slap back into reality. Dread that we'd still lose our son, because seven days from that day was just barely past 24 weeks. That was still way too early.

I nodded. I acknowledged that I heard her. I loved her. Her strength. Her determination. How much she advocated and fought for me and my son, and the care we received in the hospital. But I knew she was wrong—not about the data, but about me.

She was advising me about these numbers because that was her job, but by then it had become abundantly clear to me that we were more than the numbers and statistics. I knew we could be a story of beating the odds.

I wanted her to know that, too—not to just hear me or agree with me, but to experience it with me.

What I heard was that the odds are stacked against us, but she again didn't say 100%. That meant there are babies and women who defy the odds. That gave me hope and I knew we could continue the fight. I constantly asked myself what I could do to beat these odds and in the coming chapters you'll see what I came up with.

I made it my mission to show her what could happen when you were on Team MB. Team Miracle Baby.

I wanted her to fully experience what miracles could happen when you combine my willpower with her caring, supportive medical care, and the love and prayers from around the world.

You'll see how far we actually go, Dr. Kim.

Game on.

🌿

Hope is not a magic wand that makes everything better just because you think positively. I do not believe that hope is the cure for your pregnancy complications or your situation, nor do I believe that positive thinking will be the key to fixing everything, and you shouldn't either. So if you're thinking about past preterm deliveries or losses and wondering if you weren't hopeful enough and that's why you went through what you did, I promise you that wasn't the case.

It's about thinking about your pregnancy as a puzzle and each of these tools being pieces of that puzzle that stack the odds in your favor. Hope (and the resulting optimism) doesn't come from brute force. It comes from fully believing in your bones that you have choices, options, and control.

By asking yourself this simple question—*What can I do to beat the odds?*—you invite hope in. You allow yourself to believe that you can influence the trajectory of whatever lies ahead and you open your eyes to options that you may have never considered before. You create a plan and execute on that plan by taking action, the antidote to helplessness and hopelessness.

You're not in denial. You hear the real statistics and prognoses your doctor has laid out for you. You understand the real consequences. But you also recognize that data, research, and statistics do not define your future. You lead with the very notion that you *can* have some say in what happens next and that creates physiological changes in your body that are essential to helping heal from stress and stay pregnant.

Dr. Bruce Lipton captures this effect perfectly when he states "The moment you change your perception is the moment you rewrite the chemistry of your body."[6]

This is absolutely possible for you too.

CHAPTER 9

Impossible Decisions

Nothing is more difficult, and therefore more precious,
than to be able to decide."

—NAPOLEON BONAPARTE

You don't realize how many decisions you're required to make before your baby is born, until you are pregnant, especially if you are bringing home your first child. From different styles of cribs and rocking chairs to choosing which car seat will keep you baby the safest, there are what feels like a million choices. Add to that the feeling that you could choose wrong and hurt the baby inadvertently, and the decisions can start to feel impossible.

During a high-risk pregnancy, the stakes are even higher. Not only do you have "normal" decisions to make, but you might find yourself in the middle of making some of the hardest choices of your life related to your medical care and that of your baby during your pregnancy. It could start with choosing your OB and then later your high-risk OB. You might find it necessary to consult a specialist, like a genetics counselor, cardiologist, nephrologist, mental health counselor, or some other professional, so you have to choose the best one for you and your care.

Additionally, you might have to make decisions about whether to take medications such as antidepressants, pain relievers, or sleep supplements, or whether to do an invasive test like an amniocentesis or a surgery during pregnancy. In the most challenging of situations, you might have to make a decision about your baby's care, whether to perform surgery on the baby before or after delivery. At its most difficult, you may have to decide whether to terminate the pregnancy for any number of reasons. On top of all of this, you might find yourself making decisions about what to eat, how much to exercise, how much to rest, when to call the doctor or go to the ER if you see blood or feel contractions.

It's exhausting just to think about, let alone actually do day in and day out.

You feel the weight of the decision and worry you might make the wrong one. So you reach out to as many people as you can think of—friends, relatives, other doctors and professionals—and have them weigh in. You might even make pro-con lists to figure out how to make the best decision for you and your family, no matter how big or small that choice is. Sometimes that helps; sometimes that confuses you more.

During a high-risk pregnancy, it's possible you don't have a lot of time to make a decision. In some cases you may have days; in other cases you may have a matter of minutes. *Even* worse is that no decisions during a high-risk pregnancy can guarantee a safe, perfect outcome. The decisions you make stack the deck in your favor to help you stay pregnant, have a healthy pregnancy, and delivery a baby at term. None of them can guarantee that result, though, which makes medical decisions even more complicated and challenging during a high-risk pregnancy.

The biggest fear that I hear from clients and women I speak with is that they'll make the wrong choice and something bad will happen to the baby. They worry they'll regret a choice for the rest of their life, especially if it ends up hurting the baby, and that fear leaves them firmly planted on the fence, unable to make a decision.

I worked with one woman who couldn't decide whether to attend her best friend's wedding because she was so scared that doing so would trigger preterm labor and her baby would be born too soon. She was also terrified of losing the friendship if she stayed home and ended up delivering at term. She was able to very eloquently and successfully argue both sides of the argument for days and could not make up her mind because she was so afraid of making the wrong choice.

I also work with women after delivery, especially after a preterm birth, who are convinced that one or two decisions they made during pregnancy set the stage for the premature arrival of their little ones. The regret they live with that gnaws at them every single day and they're afraid of making the wrong choices again with their child at home.

Decision fatigue is a very real side effect of having a high-risk pregnancy, even for people who tend to otherwise be very decisive. As every decision feels so critical, sometimes with life-and-death consequences, the pressure can lead to tremendous amounts of stress, anxiety, and worry, which trickle into bodily symptoms like aches, pains, elevated blood pressure, and preterm contractions.

The good news is there is a way to make medical decisions swiftly and confidently, without having a background in medicine or science, so that you don't regret the choices you make no matter what happens going forward.

*

When we hit viability (24 weeks), it was a day of total rejoice. Everything started to change.

The conversations about my pregnancy with the medical staff seemed more upbeat and hopeful. (Granted, this was compared to "He's probably not going to make it." But at that point, every incremental change toward hope, happiness, and survival felt like a monumental shift.)

"Come on, 25!" my family cheered out as we set our eyes on the next goal: crossing 25 weeks.

The magnesium was steadily cruising through my body. My uterus had been relatively calm. My body felt surprisingly relaxed as I melted into the bed. Conversations flowed and the Travel Channel was on 24/7 to give me an escape from real life.

The next day, when I was 24 weeks and 1 day along, my uterus showed us it had other plans: I started contracting. And contracting. Despite the magnesium.

Valeria was working that night and she, along with several other nurses, rushed in. Bright lights blinded me again as they came up with a plan to figure out what to do next.

Infection was the enemy at that moment. At any sign of an infection or distress in the baby, the medical team would wave the white flag. Turn off the magnesium. Let nature take its course or get him out fast, because infection or distress meant it was no longer safe for me or baby if I stayed pregnant.

But everything checked out fine. Baby was showing no signs of distress. I had no signs of infection. No fever. No tender belly.

The uterus was just angry. Again.

We were still not friends.

Since there was no indication that delivery was imminent, did I want another bolus of magnesium? Another short, high dose of the horrible medication to try to calm my uterus down?

I hesitated.

I couldn't decide. I couldn't speak.

I was thinking clearly. I knew what was on my mind but I was spending all of my energy banishing the thoughts from my head so I couldn't actually make a choice.

It took what felt like all of the energy I had stored up in my body to nod to Sonil that I was ready for the bolus. Valeria braced me for another high dose as I prepared my body to feel like it was being hit by a bus again.

∮

There are so many reasons why we hesitate when making decisions, especially medical decisions. Not clearly understanding the choices and the related consequences is a common reason. For example, you might not understand *why* a decision about taking a particular medication needs to be made or made at this moment. Alternatively you may not understand exactly how choosing one medication over another, versus choosing no medications at all, will impact you or your baby.

This speaks to the importance of having a team of medical professionals who are on your side to explain the details to you as many times you need until you are crystal clear on what the problem is, what your choices are, and what each choice means for you and your baby going forward. I often urge clients to repeat back to their OB what they understand about their choices so their doctor can correct any misconceptions in the moment.

Often, hesitation is a sign that you're not ready to make the decision. Perhaps you're not ready to discuss delivery options because you aren't ready to accept that you will need a c-section. Or you don't want to discuss medication options because you don't want to accept that you have a complication during your pregnancy that requires medication.

Sometimes the hesitation is a sign you're feeling pressured into making a particular decision that doesn't feel right to you. For example, you might be feeling pressured to avoid an epidural when that was something you wanted to consider for yourself. So instead of committing to one or the other, you start wavering about your choices.

Relatedly, another common reason for hesitating when making a decision is not liking the options that are presented to you. For example if your doctor is telling you to choose between two medications that have side effects that don't sound comfortable for you, you may hesitate in choosing one over the other. The reality is you want neither and you worry that choosing neither isn't an option.

Understanding the underlying cause of your hesitation can help you identify your next steps, such as getting a second (or third) medical opinion, asking more questions, doing more research, or taking time to sleep on it.

One thing that you must do, no matter what the cause of the hesitation, is to manage your anxiety, because it is impossible to make a confident medical decision with high anxiety. For one, anxiety impairs how well you remember the information your doctor gives you about your situation, the choices you have, and the consequences of each choice on your health. In fact, research shows 40–80% information provided by a doctor is forgotten immediately by most patients![1] Even worse is that *of* the information that most patients remember, almost half of it is remembered incorrectly.[2] This doesn't take into account that anxiety impairs memory, so how much information you retain from your conversation with your doctor is even less than the numbers I just presented!

Yikes!

A major factor that impacts these statistics is how your doctor talks about your situation, options, prognosis, and chances of treatment success. The more worried and pessimistic they are, the less you're likely to remember everything they said.[3] This goes back to what we discussed in Chapter 2 about making sure you have doctors on your team who provide you with the real facts of your situation while still encouraging you to believe that working together can give you the best chance at beating odds.

How your prognosis and situation are framed is particularly important when you are feeling anxious because anxiety creates neurochemical changes in the brain that make you more likely to hear bad news (even if your doctor is also sharing good news) and more likely to make you assume an ambiguous situation is more negative than it actually is.[4]

You've likely experienced this yourself already. You visit your doctor and review bloodwork results. Great news: Your thyroid has leveled out but your white blood cell count is elevated. When you're already anxious about your pregnancy and the health of your baby, hearing news like that can make you zero in on the fact that your white blood cell count is higher, discounting the good news about your thyroid. Not only that, but it prevents you from hearing the details about your doctor's recommended course of action to manage your blood counts. This can further exacerbate your anxiety and keeping you stuck in an anxious loop.

Similarly, you might find that not having a clear-cut answer about what a test result means or a clear prognosis of your condition can make you assume the worst when you are anxious. For example, if your OB notices your cervix is within normal range but shorter than your last ultrasound, they might say something like, "We don't know what this means. Let's wait and see what happens."

Where does your mind go when you hear that? Likely, to the dark side, imagining worst-case scenarios, wondering why it's happening and what you did to cause it. It might lead you to Googling furiously as you're walking to your car after the appointment wondering if you should be on bed rest even if your doctor didn't mention it.

It's not just you. We all do it.

A high-risk pregnancy is a time of high stress and anxiety by the very nature of being high-risk. Also, by the very nature of being high-risk, you also have a lot of medical information to digest and likely lots of medical decisions to make. That means extra precautions have to be taken to manage your stress and worries so you can make these decisions confidently, with all of the necessary information at hand so you don't live your life with doubt or regret about the choices you make.

Most importantly, however, anxiety management is critical because what matters more than the facts, the data, and the statistics is how you feel in your body when you're considering your options and making your decision. Is your body telling you something is wrong or is your body feeling good, safe, and comfortable? What's your gut telling you is the right next step? You cannot hear that wisdom from your body if your anxiety is screaming at you.

🌿

The bolus ended after about 20 minutes, and Valeria came back, stood at the edge of my bed, and held my hand.

"What's with the hesitation?"

It wasn't said with judgment or criticism. She was simply asking a question no one else had dared ask.

"You were so certain up until this point you wanted to do everything, take every medication, throw everything at it. I want to make sure you weren't pressured into saying yes tonight."

That.

That was exactly what I needed to hear to open the doors to honesty.

As I held her hands, noticing how surprisingly soft they were considering how often she had to wash them, I felt a strength come through me to say out loud exactly what I was trying to avoid. "I wasn't hesitating about the magnesium. I'm glad we did the bolus," I said slowly. My uterus had calmed down, the contractions had stopped, and the monitors had quieted. "I just. . . ."

This was hard to say.

I was worried if I said the words out loud they would come true. But if I really paid attention to my body, the words weren't going to jinx this pregnancy. The words—the ones I was resisting so hard saying out loud—were a message from my body that knew something no one else knew at that time.

"I don't think I'm going to make it to 25 weeks," I whispered, looking at our hands.

Calm. Cool. Collected. Direct.

When I lifted my eyes to meet hers, there was a softness. An understanding. An acceptance. A realization that I had just given her information that no test, no monitor, no Magic 8 Ball would have ever been able to. Information that was from the most reliable source we had: my body.

"Every time one of my moms says that, I trust her. Because it's always true," she said, squeezing my hand.

I knew in that moment: The thread that my pregnancy was hanging on to had just gotten thinner. And flimsier. We were so much closer to the edge of the cliff than we had ever been before.

I wasn't ready to give up, but I also knew that our time was limited to throw everything at it.

At that point, I didn't care about any research study. Any statistics. Any data.

They didn't matter.

What mattered was one thing: How could I help myself stay pregnant? How could I keep my body calm? How could I stay in a place of peace so that no matter how much longer I had my son with me, he would feel that peace, that calmness, that confidence that I wanted to inject in him before he came into this world?

*

Making confident medical decisions so you don't live with doubt or regret is absolutely possible, even when you have mere minutes to make the choice. Before anything else, it requires a belief and a trust in yourself that you *can* make the right choice. Self-critical thoughts like "I don't have an MD. I can't make this decision" or "I can't understand a thing my doctor is saying. How am I ever supposed to make this decision?" have no place in the framework. Getting into the habit of being in your body and trusting your thoughts (instead of being in your head) will build the skills you need to banish those thoughts when they come creeping up.

When you're having discussions with your doctor, take notes. If you can't take notes, have someone else take them for you. Don't rely on your memory, which you've seen is deeply and easily impacted by your anxiety, to help you review the facts as you make your decision. If you can't take notes and you're by yourself at the appointment, ask for permission to record your doctor's recommendations using the voice memo app on your phone. Most doctors will be just fine with that.

During that conversation, don't be shy to ask your doctor to repeat themselves as many times as you need until you are crystal clear on what's going on, what your options are, and the impact on your health and your baby's health when choosing one of those options. If your doctor is in a rush, make another appointment or ask when you can get them on the phone to continue the discussion. If you are in a rush to make the decision like I was, keep talking and keep asking questions until you are satisfied you have the same knowledge and information that your doctor does. Again, repeat back what you heard so your doctor can correct you if you remember something incorrectly. Recitation like this also helps ensure information is stored properly in memory.

If you don't like the options your doctor has given you, seek a second opinion. If you're on hospital bed rest and can't see someone in person, many doctors offer phone consultations, so get your support system to make some calls for you until you find someone who can speak with you about your situation.

Once you feel you have all the information that you need, put the facts away. The mistake most people make when considering a medical decision is to make a pro-con list about the facts as soon as the conversation is over. They miss a critical step: identifying your personal value in this situation.

Let me explain with an example.

A high-risk OB referred her patient to me when the conversation about resuscitation came up during an appointment. Given how the pregnancy was progressing, there was a very high probability the baby was going to be born before 26 weeks, which oftentimes requires resuscitation and mechanical ventilation to help the baby breathe and survive. The stats are scary. The facts are overwhelming, and, as someone who had to make that very decision, I knew how challenging it was to make. There are considerable pros and cons on both sides, and the decision you may think you would make in a hypothetical situation may not be the one you choose when you're actually there.

It's extremely stressful and the pressure feels like the walls are closing in on you and you have nowhere to turn to escape. This woman was going back and forth on her decision. She argued both sides equally effectively. When she felt she could commit to one decision, she would burst into tears wanting to choose the other. Conversations with her partner had come to a standstill and they weren't sure what to do next.

I confirmed that she didn't need more information. She was clear about the situation and what it entailed, why this decision was on the table to begin with, why the decision needed to be made at this time, and what the impact of both choices were on her baby's future. Then I asked her the following question: "What do you want most in this particular situation?"

Naturally, in the grand scheme of things, she wanted to bring her baby home. But in this particular situation, what did she want most? Did she want her baby to have a chance at life despite how taxing it would be on her baby's body to be resuscitated? Or did she want her baby not to suffer the hardships of mechanical ventilation and extreme prematurity? Was it something else?

There are no right or wrong answers when you ask yourself this question.

We turned the tables on the internal debate she was having from the data and stats to focusing on her values. It was the first time she felt she actually had a choice. She didn't feel like she was between a rock and a hard place, being forced to choose between two really difficult options. Instead she was able to feel like she was a mother, protecting her baby, choosing the option that she felt was best for her child. That distinction created a positive feedback loop in her feelings of control and power, which elevated her mood enough to start seeing through the fog she felt she had been in. Her anxiety quieted and she was able to hear her intuition tell her what was right for her family.

This is an extreme example in which life literally hung in the balance. You may not find yourself in such a dire situation at this time, and I hope you never do! Making decisions about whether to take a particular medication, take time off of work to be on bed rest, have a sweet treat—all follow the same path that this client took. Focus on your values and allow them to guide you to the right decision for you and your family at this time.

Whatever medical decision you find yourself grappling with, the antidote to the confusion and overwhelm is taking back control. Being in control when you have to make difficult choices during your high-risk pregnancy is critical to choosing confidently and from a place of clarity, and is the only way to ensure that no matter what happens going forward, you will not regret that moment.

That control comes from leading not with the facts, but leading with your deepest, most personal values about the situation that you find yourself in and the outcome that you most desire given the circumstances.[5] From there, it's much easier to work backward to see the path you need to take to get to your ultimate goal, whatever that may be. The Ottowa Personal Decisions Guide is a fantastic free resource that can visually guide you through the steps of medical decision-making.[6]

Finally, trust your body to tell you when you've hit the right decision for you at this time. You know how that feels. Think of a time when you did something you knew you shouldn't have done but did anyway. Maybe it was taking a cookie, or five, before dinner even though you knew it would spoil your appetite. Or maybe it was hiring that employee who looked great on paper but your gut told you it was a bad move. How did you feel in your body? I've heard clients describe it as a tightness in their chest, a drop in their stomach, a racing heartbeat, or nausea. I even had one client flat-out vomit when she considered buying a house that looked great when she walked in.

Those body sensations and body memories are your clues that you were making a decision that is misaligned from your personal values and that you are possibly doing it again now.

Now turn your attention to a memory of when you made the right decision (even if it didn't seem right on paper or right to anyone else). How did that feel in your body? Clients have described this feeling as a warmth all over their body, a soaring in their chest, a lightness in their legs, like lifting a weight off their shoulders, like the elephant got up from sitting on their lungs. These are the clues, the nuggets of truth, that you want to guide you to making the right decision.

The problem most people run into is that often the decisions that make them feel like the latter are not the ones that they would have ever imagined themselves choosing. Judgments start to seep in as self-critical thoughts try to drive you off course. Making decisions by listening to these thoughts or others' thoughts on what you should do instead of your body, your instincts, and your values result in regret and a life of doubt wondering what if you chose the other option.

Remember: You can think yourself in and out of anything but your body will never, ever lie to you.

Medical decision-making is hard as it is. Doing it when another little person's life is in the balance adds tremendous pressure and can be very overwhelming. Trust that you *will* find the right solution for your family at this time. It may not be the solution you thought it would be or the one that others are telling you to make. It's your body, your baby, your pregnancy. Talk to your doctor and get all of the information you need. Then lead with your deepest values and what you want most in this situation. Finally, let your body guide you to finalizing the choice you need to make. And remember: Not choosing *is* making a choice.

CHAPTER 10

Humor and Your Pregnancy

Just imagine if we laughed more frequently,
if we had the unmitigated courage to touch each other,
it would be just the beginning of paradise – now.

—MAYA ANGELOU

Our emotional health and mental state deeply impact our bodies and our health, and the effectiveness of any stress-management strategy lies in its ability to positively change our physical health. Laughter is one of of those strategies that can do that quite effectively.

It's common knowledge that laughter is good for the health. From pain and stress relief to general improved well-being, we all know how much better we feel after a good laugh. However, laughter is so potent and powerful at improving health that cancer centers around the world have employed laughter therapy as part of their treatment programs. These programs not only help patients cope with their illness and treatment, but also show improved treatment efficacy and remission rates for those who participate.

During a health crisis like a high-risk pregnancy, laughter and humor are powerful tools to help you not only cope with intense emotions, but also turn off the stress response so your natural self-healing mechanism can help you manage your pregnancy complications. There's nothing funny about a high-risk pregnancy, but finding humor in small moments can have a long-lasting impact on your pregnancy and your overall health.

Laughter has tremendous health benefits that are far reaching into many fields of medicine. The evidence behind laughter's healing properties has been empirically proven time and time again for a wide variety of health conditions within the fields of cardiology, oncology, immunology, and even pain management. When I was researching this part of the book, I came across some amazing programs around the country that have taken this research to heart and implemented programs for laughter and humor into hospitals to help their patients heal faster.

One of my favorites is the "Laugh Wagon" that's part of the Recreational Therapy Program at Duke University's Comprehensive Cancer Center. Patients at that center are given access to materials that promote laughter, as well access to art, music, and literature, with the belief that these materials are just as critical for health and healing as medicine for their patients. Good Samaritan Hospital in Los Angeles specifically offers a "humor channel" on their TVs in patient rooms. The oncology department at St. Joseph's Hospital created a "Living Room" where patients could relax in comfortable chairs and watch funny movies as well as take part in activities such as art or reading.[1] And it works. Hospitals that have taken part in these programs have seen a significant improvement in patient health outcomes than before these programs were implemented.

Laughter is so much more than about feeling positive and happy. There are biological changes that occur in the body when we laugh. Norman Cousins, author of *Anatomy of an Illness,* found that 15 minutes of hearty laughter per day allowed him two hours of pain-free sleep despite battling a degenerative disorder of the spinal connective tissue.[2] While his account was purely anecdotal, the *New England Journal of Medicine* published his findings years later[3] because evidence for laughter as a form of healing had become incontrovertible.

Research has shown that laughter releases endorphins (our body's natural pain killer). Additionally, it stimulates the immune system, helping you fight off infections more effectively.[4] Even breastfeeding mothers and their infants get the benefit of an enhanced immune system due to laughter![5] Laughing increases blood oxygen levels, relieves muscle tension, decreases cortisol, reduces inflammation, and improves blood circulation.[6]

Essentially, laughter helps turn off the stress response and turn on the relaxation response that's designed to help you recover from the damages that stress causes. What's better? It's one of the most potent and effective tools at reducing physiological stress, and it's easy to access at any time. Though your mind (and your loved ones) can tell the difference when you laugh at something funny versus force yourself laugh, your body can't tell the difference at all. So any type of laughter helps in the same way and has the same positive effect on your endocrine, immune, and nervous systems.[7]

❧

The days on hospital bed rest had started to drag. Every hour, when the hour hand on the clock crossed 12, whoever was in the room, nurses included, would jump up and celebrate. "Woohoo!! We made it an hour!"

But the time had really started to move like molasses. Though I appreciated the celebrations, often I would be surprised, and dismayed, that only one hour had passed and it hadn't been longer.

Not having felt any direct sunlight or breathed in any fresh air for days, being confined to a horribly uncomfortable bed, and not being allowed to move took a toll on me physically and thus emotionally. My pregnancy started to feel like I was crawling uphill to the finish line miles away, parched and exhausted—with a gorilla on my back.

I knew I needed help. I needed levity. I needed something to refuel my tank. Whenever I could feel my mood dipping, feeling overwhelmed by what could happen to my son, my contractions picked up.[8] So, I'd call on my family. "Tell me a joke!" Whenever I could feel my mind going into that panicky place of "We have *how* much longer until viability?" I'd ask for a funny story. At one point someone had brought in a joke book to leave in the hospital room because they'd all run out of memorized jokes.

It gave my family something to do and helped them feel involved in keeping me happy and feeling strong. It gave me something to look forward to.

Some of the jokes were quite funny and gave me a moment of genuine belly laughter that the baby responded to also with extra punches and kicks.

Sometimes I'd laugh so hard that for a moment I forgot where I was or what was happening. I could feel the happy hormones coursing through my body. I could feel the lightness in my muscles and a joy take over my mind that helped the colors in the room look a bit brighter. I could feel my body relax. My irritable uterus would finally calm down. Even the magnesium headaches lessen in intensity.

If laughter could help a man recover from terminal heart disease, why couldn't it help me stay pregnant?

It was exactly what I, and the baby, needed. That Tuesday was no different.

We were at 24 weeks and 2 days. 24+2. One whole week since my water broke. One whole week of beating the odds. We did it!

Once the celebrations ended, I brushed my teeth, which was quite a feat considering I had to do it lying upside down. And then, I got a look on my face.

It was one Sonil hadn't seen in months. It was one that scared him. Not like the day we landed in the hospital, but because it was one that meant he was going to have to do something he really, really didn't want to do.

"Uh-oh," he said half seriously, half sarcastically. "You have an idea."
"I do!" I told him energetically.

I knew how important our surroundings are for how we feel emotionally any time in our life. If my emotions were critical to helping me stay pregnant and helping my body stay calm and helping my baby stay put, then the surroundings had to change. I couldn't get some fresh air or be around any nature or feel sunlight on my skin, but that didn't mean we couldn't do something to brighten up the space.

I asked Sonil to get my mom on the phone.

"Can you bring some construction paper and some markers and crayons when you come this morning?" She was confused but agreed. Let's be honest: Who's going to say no to the pregnant lady lying upside down, just barely passed viability, with around-the-clock headaches from the magnesium?

When she arrived a little bit later with my dad, she was relieved to see that twinkle in my eye—the one that had forced many family meetings when I was a child and that had been the source of the craziest of ideas for vacations or restaurants to try.

Let's make Moroccan turkey for Thanksgiving this year!
How about we go to the Galapagos Islands for summer vacation?
Who wants to try a fire-eating class?

All shot down. It never stopped me from trying, though, and this day was no different.

"We need more positive messages all around. Wherever I look, I want to see something positive because that helps me stay calm and I know that will inspire this baby stay put," I declared.

They were listening intently as I spoke with a confidence and authority that I hadn't had in many weeks. It was a relief for them, too, to see me in my element.

"Can you all draw pictures for him telling him to hold on in there?"
"Oh no . . . ," Sonil said, as he sank into the sofa, shaking his head.

My mom's face turned red from laughter. She asked if I really wanted *her* to draw something, knowing her drawing skills were on par with her ability to fly.

My dad was the first to sit down with a marker and a paper and get going. He's our resident artist, so he loved the idea. And, who's he to say no to his daughter, right?

My brother and best friend joined soon after and I asked them to do the same thing. They also responded with eye rolls and groans. "You know I can't draw!" my best friend said to me.

"I know. That's the point!" I said, laughing.

The sight of seeing some of my favorite people in the room engaging in a creative activity that was meant to change the feel of the sterile hospital room was life-altering.

I felt the energy and the buzz in the room reverberate throughout my body. I was relaxed. So was my uterus.

Their laughs and hoots as they peeked over at each other's drawings, ones I couldn't see because I was upside down facing the ceiling, made my heart swell.

This is the family you're going to be born into. We're weird. We laugh. We do silly things. I can't wait for you to be a part of this. But please, hang on for a little while longer, MB.

My dad was the first to be done, and he proudly sauntered over to the side of my bed and held the picture up for me to see.

He had written a nickname he wanted to give the baby: *jadoo*, meaning magic. My dad had been moved to see how much this little person had overcome and survived through this pregnancy. "He's just magic," he'd said so many times.

I loved it.

Until I saw what was underneath. This picture, which was supposed to be of a baby with a newborn hat, looked like a wrinkly middle-aged man who had left his life as a professional thug.

"Apparently I'm going to give birth to a 55-year-old mobster," I said wiping the tears from my eyes as I laughed with the rest of my family.

We were so loud our nurse came in to see what the commotion was. She took one look and was intrigued by the project. She took time to see everyone's drawings, sometimes being very careful to be polite with her reactions.

When she left, several other nurses came by to see what we were up to. My family was busy drawing and showing me their creations.

One picture looked like a chimp hanging from a tree with a big "Hold on!" sign above it.

One looked like *Mrs. Doubtfire's* face mask after the garbage truck had driven over it.

They were hilarious. And absolutely perfect.

"One last thing," I told my brother after they'd taped the pictures to the wall where I could see them. I wanted the overwhelming message in the room to be "hang on!" So my brother cut up small pieces of paper and, on these 1 inch by 2 inch slips, wrote "Hang on MB."

Hang on, Miracle Baby.

The rest of the family joined in, and within a few minutes, we had about 40 slips of paper all over the room. On the IV stand. On the lights. On the clock. On the sink. On the frame of the TV.

Everywhere you looked, there was that message—the only message I wanted from that point until the end. And everywhere I turned, there was something to laugh at.

Though I saw OBs from Dr. Edwards's practice every single day, I hadn't seen Dr. Kim for several days. This was a good thing because it was a testament to how stable things had become. I wasn't contracting very much, and I was feeling well emotionally and physically. Things had calmed down. At last!

Finally, on a Thursday night, she walked in at 9 p.m. I couldn't believe how late she was working. She looked tired, but anyone could see this job wasn't work for her; it's her life blood. It came through in the way she always spoke to me.

I wanted to give her a hug and thank her for being on my medical team.

I also wanted to gloat a little, but I didn't have a chance to. She looked around the room, took in the signs and hilarious pictures my family had created and looked at me. "You're still here!" she said with much warmth in her voice.

Yes, I was! I beat the odds. I'd stayed pregnant for nine days, something more than 75% of women don't typically experience after their water breaks.

We'd done it!

She didn't have to say any more. She smiled at us and, through her tired eyes, I knew we'd converted her. She had officially joined Team MB, Team Miracle Baby—a team that didn't follow the statistics.

We made a plan to come off the magnesium at 25 weeks because being on for that long wasn't good for me or the baby. But Sonil and I wanted a few more days to cross into the next week, which could give him a significantly better chance of survival than if he were born sooner.

She agreed. We all smiled. We were all—each and every one of us—so hopeful for the future. The most we'd been since I landed in the hospital exactly two weeks prior.

We were making miracles.

🌿

Laughter is potent and powerful and helps you feel more positively during a medical crisis like a high-risk pregnancy. Physically, it relaxes your body and allows your nervous, immune, and endocrine systems to come back into balance.

By infusing laughter into your every day, you can experience long-lasting effects on your health through the postpartum period and beyond. In my mind, it needs to be an essential part of prenatal care, especially during a complicated pregnancy. Laughter yoga is a fantastic way to stay healthy especially if you have activity restrictions or are on bed rest. Several of my clients have experienced a decrease in preterm contractions and blood pressure when they've practiced laughter yoga. One of them even had her partner join her in her laughter yoga sessions, which was a fantastic way for them to bond while she was on bed rest and reconnect outside of the stress of her pregnancy. (To download a free visual guide on how to practice laughter yoga, visit pbres.pregnancybrainbook.com.)

However, I do want to be careful about overstating the effects of laughter. To think that laughter alone can cure you of your pregnancy complications or that it can be a substitute for traditional medical care is erroneous. Laughter is a supplemental tool that is just as important as prenatal care with your board-certified OB-GYN or MFM.

I also want to acknowledge that sometimes there's nothing to laugh about. Sometimes, you're so down, so discouraged, or so overwhelmed by the reality that lies ahead of you that you can't get yourself to laugh. No number of online memes or stand-up comedy routines on Comedy Central get that belly laugh going.

If that's your reality right now, that's okay. Don't fight it. Laughter is not possible all the time and it is not always effective. If laughing feels challenging, accept that. Tune into your body to find out what it needs instead of laughter to help you turn on your self-repair mechanism, your relaxation response. Ask yourself *"What does my body need?"* Notice where you're holding onto tension or discomfort and then give your body what it needs to relieve that. But when you're ready and feel like you can take a shot at laughing again, give it a try. It's potent, it's powerful, it's free, and it's always available to you to help you heal from the physical and emotional stress you're under during this pregnancy.

CHAPTER 11

Thriving on Love

"You loved me before seeing me;
You love me in all my mistakes;
You will love me for what I am."

—LUFFINA LOURDURAJ

When I began writing this book, my primary goal was to show you, the reader, how much power you have within your body to protect your baby. With resources built into your body naturally to help you repair from the hormonal, muscular, and cellular damage that stress causes, your body is designed to do whatever it can to help you stay pregnant and keep your baby safe. It's mind-blowing and changes the way that I experienced my body and the way that I now understand health, especially reproductive health. I hope you have really felt the depths of the power that lies in your body, too, to turn the helplessness into control, anxiety into peace, and sadness into confidence.

However, this is not the whole story. You can do everything right—have access to the best medical care, eat well, exercise as allowed by your body and OB, get enough sleep, prioritize activating the relaxation response to help your body heal and repair from stress—and still experience some of the biggest heartbreak a parent can have: a baby born too soon with weeks or months in the NICU. Or a baby whom you have to carry with you in your heart instead of in your arms.

It happens. It's unfair. It's life-shattering. It's not your fault.

There's no way to know exactly how your pregnancy will play out, but there is one more thing that you can do for yourself and your baby when you're pregnant as you fight to give your little miracle a chance at life. It's the one thing that no one else on this planet do, not even your doctor or your partner. It's the one thing that your baby needs from you and you only. . . .

Love. Deep, profound, life-altering maternal love from the bottom of your heart every moment of every day.

I say this not because I think you don't love your baby, but because during a high-risk pregnancy it's very easy to dissociate from your body and pregnancy, and forget about this important aspect of health. It's easy to experience your body as different, separate and distinct from who you are as a person.

The evidence of that is how you talk about your situation and conceptualize what's happening.

I've heard from so many clients comments like:

"I've always been so successful but my body is failing us."

"I'm a strong person. Why is my body so weak?"

"I'm usually so on top of things and so put together. My body is falling apart."

"This pregnancy is so messed up."

Or women swing the other direction and turn their complications into a part of their identity, feeling like they *are* their pregnancy:

"I'm broken."

"I'm a failure."

"I'm weak."

And yet for others, it's not something they say but something they feel. Recently, a client shared with me that she had stopped thinking about her baby when she was on hospital bed rest because she didn't want to be reminded of her, or how scary the situation was and how close she was to losing this baby. So she tried not to get attached.

All of these efforts are in the name of self-preservation.[1] You're protecting your heart from breaking in case something bad happens. If you've experienced preterm delivery[2] or loss in the past, you're bracing yourself for the heartbreak you've already experienced.[3] It's a completely understandable reaction, though it does impact your ability to bond with your baby.[4]

The disembodied, detached experience increases emotional and physical distress during pregnancy, which we've seen throughout the book can become risk factors for many different types of pregnancy complications. Reconnecting with their body and bonding with their baby is one aspect of the work I focus on with my clients. Together we work to rebuild confidence in her body and reshape her core identity (which has often changed because of past experiences of infertility, loss, and/or prematurity).[5]

Your attachment to your pregnancy, your body, and, most importantly, your baby has tremendously powerful healing properties that can turn off your stress response and turn on the relaxation response. Through the "love hormone" called oxytocin, research has shown shifts and positive changes to your immune system and endocrine system, as well as a decrease in stress hormones and inflammation.[6] The love you have for your baby helps you and helps your baby during your high-risk pregnancy.

Practicing mindfulness,[7] body-focused exercises like biofeedback to help you stay connected to your body, and visualization have all been shown to lower anxiety, elevate confidence, and increase prenatal attachment with your baby. They've also shown to increase blood flow to the baby by way of reducing inflammation and stress hormones in the body.[8] (For a description of exercises to try, please see Appendix A and Appendix B.)

It all comes down to believing that your love matters, not just emotionally but physically, for you and your baby, trusting that it is an important aspect of your prenatal care during a high-risk pregnancy, and then doing what you can to stay connected to that bond and deep love for your baby, even when you're scared to get too attached.

*

The following day started out as any other. Celebrations for getting through another night. For making it to Friday.

TV to pass the time.

Crossword puzzles and trivia quizzes to stay busy.

Knock-knock jokes to keep me laughing.

My mom had sent a tuna sandwich, which I had been craving, with my dad, my babysitter for the early afternoon.

I could only get down half before I lost my appetite. No one was worried. I hadn't stood up in 10 days. I had been lying with my head below my feet for 15 days. It was only natural my appetite would be diminished.

Shift change for us happened when new nurses came on and also when new babysitters for me arrived.

At four o'clock, my dad's shift ended and my mom came to take over. They talked between themselves about what happened all morning, about my mood, and about what my mom should expect.

"It's a quiet day," my dad told her. "I'll see you tonight."

My mom came in, gave me a hug, and asked how I was feeling. I reassured her I was feeling fine. A little tired, but otherwise calm.

Not even 10 minutes after my dad left, it all changed.

Tightness in my back that made me squirm. Contractions in my belly that made me ask my mom to call the nurse urgently. *Something was wrong.*

I had had six weeks of contractions up until that point. I was familiar with them. I knew what they felt like.

They didn't feel like this. This was different. *Something was wrong.*

The nurse came and checked my temperature.

No fever.

She checked my belly.

No tenderness.

She checked my son's heartbeat.

All normal.

"Something's not right," I told her.

That was her cue to escalate.

She went to page the on-call OB, and by the time she came back I was wriggling and moaning in discomfort. Nothing really hurt that bad physically but I was vocalizing my fears.

Something was wrong.

My mom decided to call Sonil and tell him to come to the hospital. She stepped away to call him, and when she came back the nurse was obsessively checking my temperature and baby's heartbeat. *Something was wrong.*

"Stay with me, okay?" I whispered to my mom. She held on to my hand and reassured me with her eyes and her nods that she wasn't going anywhere.

The on-call OB ran in with my nurse close behind. The OB was the same one who admitted me to the hospital 15 days earlier.

She checked me and the room went quiet.

"Why does it hurt so much?" I asked the OB. It didn't actually hurt very much at all. It was uncomfortable and contractions were strong, but it didn't hurt. I just needed her to stay the words.

"Because you're in labor." I finally opened my eyes to look at her and she said quietly, "It's time to have the baby."

Instantly, the room changed. Nurses came charging in. The sound level in the room increased tenfold as instructions were being flung from across the room to the teams of people that were there.

My internal alarms started ringing. Calmness? Gone. Relaxation response? Very much off.

Lizard brain. Grizzly bear. Run.

I had no idea how to have a baby. I never took any child-birthing classes. How was I supposed to know how to get this baby out? I didn't know how to deliver. I didn't know how to breathe. What was I supposed to do again?

My mind immediately went to Joey. The kidney stone! Ross was yelling, "Push!!"

Thank goodness for Friends!

But I wasn't ready to push yet. I wasn't ready for this to be happening.

I felt my mom hold onto my right hand and arm. I felt Aliya, my delivery nurse, hold onto my left arm. I saw the bright lights turn on and I realized I couldn't deny this anymore.

This is it.

These were my last moments with my son. This was the last time I could let him get some strength from me and my body. The last time I could give him a feeling of peace directly from me.

I closed my eyes and tuned everything out.

The sounds became muffled. I was just there with my son, my little miracle baby. I pictured the last ultrasound I had of him. The 3D picture with his hands by his face, his little knob of a nose and his tiny, pointed chin.

He was perfect.

I focused on that image and nothing else. I allowed that image and the love I felt for him to fill my body, trusting he could feel it too o he could have a final few moments of tranquility.

"Okay, push." I heard my OB's distant voice.

I stayed focused on that ultrasound picture. My strong, perfect little boy. His perfect little nose. His tiny little hands. My miracle baby. My MB.

I took a deep breath and let out a sound, not for physical pain. It was the sound of the pain of my heart completely shattering.

In less than a count of three, the pressure was gone. My belly was empty.

He was born.

My pregnancy was over.

The NICU team grabbed him and ran him to the unit to resuscitate him before Sonil had made it to the room. He'd missed the delivery.

Cramping from the pitocin (to help my uterus contract back down) made me open my eyes. When I looked up, the first person I saw was Dr. Kim. She was standing next to the delivering OB, her face expressing every emotion I couldn't feel yet.

"I'll go find Dad. I know what he looks like," she said quietly as she left the room.

There was some pain from the cramping. It was nothing I couldn't tolerate. But I didn't want to feel a thing. I wanted to be numb. Devoid of all feeling. I asked for pain killers because I knew the moment that the shock faded, the emotional pain would be unbearable.

It took almost three hours for me to acclimate to sitting upright again without feeling lightheaded or like I was about to pass out. After having been upside down for 15 days, the room looked foreign to me from a sitting position.

This was our battleground, where the most epic fight had taken place, with our nurses and doctors, and with prayers and love from around the world.

I saw the aftermath. Our belongings thrown to the side to make room for the delivery and the NICU teams.

The bed that had become my home, no more a safe haven of hope.

Once I could sit up for several minutes without fainting, my nurse got me in a wheelchair and took me to the NICU, his new home, to meet my son for the first time. We had no idea how long he would survive. If he would survive. It was even more excruciating than the unknowns of my pregnancy.

She pulled me up beside his isolette (the plastic box that was keeping him warm). I saw his tiny body. His little knob of a nose. His tiny, pointed chin. Covered in tubes and wires.

He was perfect.

"You fight like hell," I whispered to him through the plastic box. "Please. Fight like hell."

Aliya wheeled me back to the mother-baby unit, where everyone was waiting for me and Sonil.

The room was small. Again. The same type of room I was in before.

A reminder that I was one of *those* moms—the ones who didn't have a baby in room with me.

We'd amassed *a lot* of "stuff" over the previous days. More flowers. More cards. Lots of signs with messages to my son to hang on, which he did until it wasn't safe anymore. He had gotten the message and he hung on for dear life until it was time.

"What's his name?" my mom asked when I got comfortable in bed and dried my tears.

"Vihaan," I told her softly.

First light of dawn. New beginnings.

❦

It might seem obvious that it's important to bond with your baby in utero, but I've personally experienced and seen with my clients how challenging that is when anxiety is high and fears about losing the baby are very real. That says nothing about you as a mother and everything about how challenging the situation is that you're in.

A study was conducted in the 1970s with rhesus monkeys who were raised in lab. They had access to a "mother"—basically wires that were molded into the shape of a monkey and covered in warm, fuzzy material. Next to this "mother" was another monkey made of wire, without the fuzzy material, that had a bottle filled with milk. While the monkey would go to the "mother" with milk when hungry, it spent most of its time with the mother that provided warmth. The hypothesis was that mothers provide more value with their warmth than by nutrition and that a child will bond with the mother who provides warmth not the one who provides just nourishment.[9]

I thought of this study frequently during my high-risk pregnancy, because it reminded me of my role in my son's development and his life. It's why I'm sharing it with you right now to remind you of your role in your baby's life:

You are more than an incubator or a vessel for your baby. You are a whole, complete woman who is capable of providing your child something that is essential for his or her growth and development in utero that no one else can provide. Your love for your baby is an invaluable and essential component of your prenatal care and what is required for you to stay pregnant during your high-risk pregnancy.

Does that mean that you didn't love your baby enough with previous losses or preterm deliveries? Absolutely not.

It means that you have a choice going forward to shift how you conceptualize and experience your pregnancy in a way I'm certain your doctor is not considering when it comes to a prenatal care plan. I know for a fact that when you allow yourself to believe that your love is critical to growing a healthy baby, and you allow that love to course through your blood, physiological changes happen. You relax. Your body relaxes. Your baby thrives. You start to feel a sense of control and power about how you can help yourself and your baby as you fight to make it as close to term as you possibly can.

Here's a simple way to try it right now. Sit comfortably and close your eyes. Put your hands on your belly. (If that triggers any feelings of guilt, shame, anxiety or fear, put your hands on your heart.) Imagine a light coming from your heart that covers your entire body, from your shoulders and arms, down to your feet and toes. Visualize that light surrounding your baby, who is nestled comfortably in your belly. Imagine that light protecting your baby, surrounding her with the nourishment he or she needs to grow and thrive and to be at peace. Clients have reported this exercise bringing tears to their eyes. Allow them to flow. These are tears of release, creating space in your body for repair and healing.

Staying connected with your body and believing in the power of your love helps you have a healthy high-risk pregnancy and it also helps with healing postpartum. When you look back on this time and the journey you've been on, whether you deliver preterm, hold this baby in your heart, or take your baby home after a full-term delivery, you will know you did everything you possibly could to give your baby a chance at life.

No one loves your baby as much as you do. Trust that this love is exactly what your baby needs as you fight to give him or her a strong start to life.

The Power of You

*The body always leads us home . . . if we can simply learn to trust
sensation and stay with it long enough for it to reveal appropriate
action, movement, insight, or feeling.*

—PAT OGDEN

Often when research in the field of mind-body medicine, lifestyle
medicine, and psychoneuroimmunology is presented, the pushback
is around the distinction between *curing* and *healing*. We tend to
use these words interchangeably when in fact they are very different
in many ways.

OB-GYN and mind-body expert Dr. Lissa Rankin sums it up
perfectly when she states, "You can be cured without being healed
and you can be healed without being cured."[1] The goal of this
book is not to teach you tools that will cure you of your pregnancy
complications. It would be wholly inaccurate for me to say that
anything I've shared in this book will cure you of a medical problem
that you are currently facing during your high-risk pregnancy.

The tools that I've shared throughout this book are designed to help you heal. They are designed to activate a natural repair system that's built into your body whose sole purpose is to help you stay pregnant and help your baby stay safe for as long as possible. The impact of turning on this relaxation response helps you regain control during a time when you feel helpless and guide you toward feeling whole and complete again once your baby is born. What I know for a fact is that when my clients have approached their prenatal health from a place of overcoming a challenge, having hope and believing that they can influence their pregnancy journey, miraculous changes to their health happen. They can happen for you, too.

Decades of research have shown this to be true for countless complications that are impacted by stress, including:

- Preeclampsia,
- Gestational hypertension,
- Gestational diabetes,
- Placental abruption,
- Preterm cervical shortening or incompetent cervix,
- Uterine irritability or preterm contractions,
- Preterm labor,
- Intrauterine growth restriction, and
- Poor blood flow to baby.

You may not be cured from your complications. As you've seen, I was far from cured from any of mine. But you have everything to gain from taking charge of your health, reclaiming your body, and getting back in the driver's seat of your pregnancy to find the solutions that will help turn on the natural self-healing mechanism in your body to help you stay pregnant as long as possible—whether that's a few days, a few weeks, or all the way to term.

Research has shown that our bodies are far more powerful and robust than modern medicine has us believe. We often underestimate our strengths and overestimate our weaknesses, feeding into the belief that we are at the mercy of medicine and luck without having a say about the trajectory of the pregnancy going forward. We are not nearly as helpless during a medical crisis like a high-risk pregnancy as we think and are told.

Relatedly, believing that you can influence your health by making confident medical decisions, and that your body is designed to help you stay pregnant and grow a healthy baby, is critical to the health of your pregnancy. Trust that your body has a built-in self-repair system that you can turn on at any time. Open your mind about what's possible during your pregnancy, even if you have complications. Allow yourself to shift your beliefs from the impossible to the possible, from helplessness to control. As Henry Ford said, "Whether you think you can, or you think you can't— you're right."

To be able to make these mental shifts so that you can feel the positive changes to your body physiologically requires the right team to surround you. If you have a doctor, nurses, and specialists who view your complications as obstacles that can be overcome, who recognize that statistics are just likelihoods and not crystal balls, and who place value on your expertise of your body, you're far more likely to have a positive response to whatever the treatment protocol they recommend than if none of these factors are in place.

Similarly, surrounding yourself with supportive friends and family is critical to your emotional and physical health. It's easy to isolate yourself during a high-risk pregnancy when you realize how few people truly understand the challenges you face. Keep an open mind about who might be able to support you. In many cases, the best support can come from the most unlikely sources— acquaintances you reconnect with, a coworker you barely talk to, or new friends you meet online or in support groups.

Despite all of this, remember to be realistic about the mind-body impact. Even the most hopeful, positive, optimistic attitudes are no guarantee of a particular positive outcome, but these emotional states can create the right environment in your body for medical treatments to be more effective and for your self-repair system to help you heal from the damages of stress. Your goal is not to cure yourself of the complications you're facing, but to give your body the best chance to help yourself stay pregnant as long as possible, which relying on the mind-body connection helps you do.

Your body is always communicating with you and it never lies. By quieting the mental chatter influenced by anxiety, grief, or guilt, you can listen to that little voice in the back of your head that's calm, cool, collected, and direct that's always telling you what your body needs. Physical symptoms are your body's way of sending you a message that will clue you in on what you need to do to help yourself during your pregnancy. We often ignore these messages because our anxiety is too high or because we don't like what the message is telling us. Trust that by listening to your body and the early warning whispers, you can get the best care you need as early as possible to help you and your baby the most effectively during your high-risk pregnancy.

Despite doing everything you can, there are still things during a high-risk pregnancy that are out of your control. You are not at fault for the complications you have, the circumstances around your baby's delivery, or what happens after you give birth. It's easy to get caught up in self-blame; however when viewed through the lens of compassion without judgment, a high-risk pregnancy can afford invaluable insight on how to support your body to help you stay pregnant.

There is so much more research to be done; there's more data to be collected to show the depth of the mind-body connection and its power in helping women with high-risk pregnancies and lowering the preterm birth rate. Our work has just begun. However, your journey to experiencing a miracle can begin immediately. By opening your mind to a new way of conceptualizing stress, pregnancy, your reproductive health, and what it really means to have "pregnancy brain," you can help yourself have a healthy pregnancy starting now.

As I sit here, reflecting on one of the scariest times of our life, when Vihaan's life hung in the balance for so many months, it's easy to wonder whether stress caused him to come early. Still, to this day, my mind goes there. But I know for a fact the answer to that is no. Stress does not *cause* any of these complications on its own for any of us.

Could I have stayed pregnant a little bit longer, maybe a few days to cross into 25 weeks or a few weeks to cross into the third trimester, if I had been able to receive the proper mind-body support for stress management earlier in my pregnancy? We'll never know, and that's an unknown I will live with for the rest of my life.

What I do know is that relying on my relaxation response was a critical piece of the puzzle that bought us 15 more days at the end of my pregnancy. I also know that when he was born, it was because my body knew it was time. Had he stayed in any longer, my health and his health would have been in jeopardy. I do trust, now, that my body knew it was time and delivering at 24+5 given everything that had happened in the pregnancy thus far, was the best chance that both he and I had at surviving. That gives me the peace I need to heal from that traumatic time of our life.

That is the peace I want for you, too.

🌿

Breakfast was done. Two rounds of pumping were finished. Showers were taken. Bags were packed.

And then the phone rang.

My heart stopped. Sonil froze. We looked at each other and took in the sound. The call we had waited so long for.

I ran into the home office, which had turned into a storage dump. "Hello?"

My voice was shaking. My hands were shaking more. I don't even remember if I was breathing.

"Mrs. Deshpande? Your son is ready to come home."

I have tears writing that. Still. Right now. I'm sitting here in tears.

I can hear her soft, sweet voice on the other end of the line. I can feel my heart swell as I heard the words we'd been dying to hear. For months, these were words we weren't sure we'd ever hear. Words that changed our life completely.

Today was the day. Today was homecoming day.

Vihaan had been in the NICU for 109 days, a mere blip on the radar for most 24-weekers. To tell you what happened in those 109 days would make this book rival *War and Peace* in length. Suffice to say for now, it was hard. Horribly, gut-wrenchingly, life-alteringly hard. There were moments in the NICU I wouldn't wish even my worst enemies experience.

He was the sickest baby in the NICU when he was born. So sick, he had a personal bodyguard—just one nurse, watching over him for the first few weeks. She had no other patients. No other cases. Just him, because he was so fragile.

Over those 109 days, we watched him grow and thrive. He learned how to maintain his body temperature so he could come outside of the isolette and out into an open-air crib, a moment I'll never forget because I could touch him whenever I wanted. He learned how to eat, how to grow, and eventually how to get through each day without his heart rate dropping or his oxygen levels crashing.

And finally, that incredibly special day was here: the day he could say goodbye to the hospital, breathe fresh air for the first time, and finally go home.

When we got onto the freeway, reflexively Sonil and I sighed.

A sigh of relief. Of release. Of memories of being on that road, that fateful day at 22+4 in pitch black, not knowing that was the last time I would be pregnant at home. Not knowing what tumultuous, horribly heartbreaking moments lay ahead of us.

Not knowing that a miraculous day like this day could happen.

I looked out the window as we made the trek to the hospital one last time, and it struck me how the whole world looked exactly the same: people heading to work and dropping off children at school. Frustrated drivers cutting each other off to beat the morning commute. Green hills looking strong, majestic, and beautiful, bringing a sense of peace just like the day we transferred that one, little, three-day embryo.

But our entire world had changed.

Over the previous year, our hearts had shattered in many places. I wasn't sure we could fully heal. I still had physical scars from the epic fight for Vihaan's life in the last 15 days of my pregnancy. I still do, to this day. We have memories of moments that most parents can't begin to imagine their children going through. We have fears because of what we'd witnessed can happen to a human at the edge of life.

Our homecoming day had so much history behind it. Its meaning and the significance and magnitude of it were beyond what we could explain in words.

We pulled into the parking lot, unloaded our gear, and made our way through two security checkpoints to our little guy, who was waiting for us. Who had no idea how big the outside world was that was waiting for him.

I walked over to his little bassinet, which had been his home. Looking into his big, beautiful eyes, I smiled as I finally got to unhook the leads that had connected his body to the hospital for 109 days.

I gently removed the stickers from his chest that had monitored his life since the moment he was born.

The nurse turned off the monitors that we had watched so intently for months as we prayed for oxygen levels to bounce back or his heart rate to even out.

I put him in the outfit I had picked out weeks before in anticipation of this day.

Orange shirt. Blue pants. Blue socks. Striped hat.

We took so many photos of the machines, his crib, the hospital.

As much as I hated to admit it, this had been his first home. This was where he grew and became the baby who was strong enough to come home. I wanted memories of all of it to show him someday how much he had overcome.

We said our goodbyes, and as I carried his bags of medications and supplies, Sonil carried this tiny human in his car seat out of the unit, into the hallway, and to the lobby of the hospital.

He placed the carseat on a bench, where I sat, taking in my miracle child seeing sunlight for the first time through the large window that opened to the atrium.

I kept looking down the hallway expecting a nurse to come running, asking us to bring him back. I kept eyeing the security guard who was sitting near us, wondering if I was giving off a guilty vibe for child kidnapping.

Was it really time? Was he really ours to take home?

Sonil pulled up the car to the front door and it hit me. It took my breath away and I stood for a moment, frozen.

This is our moment. This is the moment we never got throughout the pregnancy.

The monumental moment that changed us forever. The moment we could celebrate without an asterisk. The moment that made our hearts explode.

Pure and simple, it was the happiest moment of our lives.

From the outside, you'd never know what this moment really meant. We looked like any other couple, unsure of what to do with this baby, completely terrified (and convinced) we were going to drop him somehow.

We looked like any first-time parents, with *way* too much gear for a baby who needed nothing but food, shelter, and love.

We looked like any other brand-new family of three, ready for our new adventure together.

After the slowest 30-mile drive in the history of driving, Sonil, Vihaan, and I arrived home. Sonil, in his favorite tan sweater and jeans, carried the carseat up the stairs from the garage to the living room. I followed behind in gray pants and a black jacket.

My vision had become a reality.

It took my breath away. I wanted to savor it. Every last second of it. This was our moment.

Several days earlier, Sonil sat next to me while I pumped milk for Vihaan. We knew Vihaan was coming home soon but the hospital staff had yet to tell us a definitive date.

I was playing The Sims on my iPod. (Next adventure: get a smartphone.)

He looked at me with tears in his eyes. "You did this. You stayed pregnant just long enough for him to survive. You advocated for him in the NICU. You got him the best care. You did this. I hope you can see that."

I knew in my head I did everything I could. I had squeezed every last drop of water out of the sponge that was my pregnancy by helping my body stay relaxed and helping my uterus keep him in until the very last moment. I knew in my head that, had I stayed pregnant longer, the infection that had developed in my body would have hurt us both, or worse.

But I also knew that there was a lot of healing left to do, because the guilt was still very palpable. The guilt had made a home in my heart.

We still had a long road with Vihaan. Whenever he came home, we knew it would be the end of one chapter and the beginning of the next: caring for a micropreemie, a medically fragile child. It would be a whole other marathon with hurdles I didn't yet know.

But in that moment, I allowed Sonil's words to sink in. I didn't believe them yet fully, but I trusted him that he saw something more clearly than I could see. For as trusting as I was of my gut when it came to my pregnancy and to Vihaan's health in the NICU, it was completely unreliable when it came to judging my role in helping Vihaan survive.

So, I put my faith in him. I trusted that he wasn't just saying that because he had to or because he had nothing else to say.

He was saying it because it was true. It was my job to learn how to believe that.

Calm. Cool. Collected. Direct.

❧

To call this phase of our life and the work I've done since a learning experience is the understatement of a lifetime. My eyes have been opened to the power of the human body, the power of the mind, and how deep that well of strength goes when you have to fight for your child.

If there's one thing I've taken away from the madness that was bringing this little boy home and that I hope you take away from reading this book, it's this:

I wish you didn't have to be so strong. I wish this journey wasn't so hard for you, too. I wish that with all my might.

The hope you're so desperately searching for, the answers and the predictions of the future that you so desperately want, aren't going to come from what your doctor tells you or how an ultrasound looks or any statistics anyone quotes for you. They're going to come from realizing that your body holds the answers. Your body knows what's happening, what's going on, and what it needs to help you stay pregnant. Your body knows how to protect your baby and your body from the effects of stress. It's going to come from allowing yourself to accept that you have more power than you realize to help yourself stay pregnant even when everything feels like it is falling apart.

I don't know what will happen in your pregnancy, when you'll deliver, or what will happen to your baby. If there was a crystal ball, I would send it to you right now. But know that you are so much stronger than you feel. You have more control than you're being made to believe.

Use it to build a medical team of doctors and nurses who love you and believe in you, who will tell you the truth no matter how hard it is to hear, and who will then fight with you and for you until the very end, no matter what odds are stacked against you. Do your homework and speak up when something feels wrong, because you are your baby's best advocate and loudest voice. Surrender to the uncertainty and allow your body to do what it can, the best it can, for as long as it can. Trust that your body knows what it needs to help you stay pregnant and follow its lead.

The hope that comes from experiencing how much your body changes physically when you tap into the power of the mind shines bright and will give you the strength, the force, the fortitude to fight on for one more hour. One more day.

Take charge of your health. Tap into your inner mama bear, be unapologetically loud about your concerns, and keep searching for the people to add to your team who can help you. Allow yourself to believe anything is possible and that miracles can happen for you too. Hold on firmly to the knowledge that you have more control and more power than you realize to influence your pregnancy and unleash that power to allow for amazing things to happen for you and your baby.

You are more than a number. More than your diagnosis. More than a statistic.

I hope you can feel those words in your bones today and every day for the rest of your pregnancy.

Take it one day, one step at a time, and prepare yourself for miracles to take your breath away.

Relaxation: Letting Your Body Lead

Physiological relaxation is at the core of having a healthy pregnancy, especially if you're experiencing pregnancy complications. It turns on the self-repair mechanism to help your body recover from damages of stress, whether it's stress from pain, lack of sleep, anxiety, low mood, loneliness, guilt, grief, or any other type of stress your body is under. Recovery allows your body's hormonal, neurological, and immune systems to fall back into the delicate balance that's required to have a healthy pregnancy.

Knowing *how* to turn on this relaxation response is dependent on getting out of your head and into your body. How many times have you told yourself, "I'm not tired" or "It doesn't hurt much," trying to convince yourself that things are not as bad as they seem? We've all done it! We can talk ourselves in and out of anything, but our bodies never lie. Unfortunately, learning to listen to our bodies and their signals is not a skill most of us learn, so it's okay if it doesn't come naturally to you right away.

The good news is that it's not difficult to do. With daily practice you can learn how to turn off the chatter in your head and start listening to the only source of truth about your health: your body. So before you try any more breathing techniques or guided meditations, prenatal yoga classes, or visualizations, start here to learn what *exactly* your body needs so you can choose the right tool and exercise to help. Below, I outline the three-step process on how to reconnect with your body gently and safely so you can let your body lead you to healing from stress and a healthier pregnancy.

Step 1: Feel with your hands.

Every day, choose an item around the house. Hold it in your hands, close your eyes, and spend 30–60 seconds describing the physical sensation of holding that object.

The purpose of this exercise is to reconnect you with your body. Consider it like a warm-up jog before you start your full run. You'll know you've reconnected with your body effectively when the thoughts in your mind quiet or disappear completely. You might notice other parts of your body relaxing slightly, such as your shoulders dropping or slower breathing. Doing this every day, multiple times per day, helps create a new habit of learning to listen to your body while quieting your thoughts.

This is also an excellent tool to come back to you if you notice your anxiety rising—for example, in the doctor's waiting room, as your OB is reviewing test results with you, or as you're waiting for the call from your doctor to know what to do next. The sooner you can get out of your head and into your body, the quicker you can turn on the relaxation response.

Step 2: Build body intelligence.

Once you've mastered Step 1 (and with daily practice, it doesn't take long to master), turn your attention to your body to gain clarity on how it's feeling in the moment. Pay attention to sensations such as pain, tightness, and soreness, as well as sensations that feel good to you.

As you notice these parts of your body, be sure to describe in detail *how* that sensation feels. For example, if you have pain in your calf, describe the pain as shooting, aching, dull, bruised, and so on. These words are clues and signals that your body frequently uses to get your attention. The more aware you are of them, the faster you'll realize what your body is trying to tell you.

There are two effective ways to complete this step. Choose the one that best resonates with you: journaling or body scan.

Journaling

Every day, multiple times per day, answer the following journal prompt:

How is my body feeling right now?

Where is my body tight and holding tension?

What does the tension feel like?

Where is there pain?

What does the pain feel like?

Where in my body do I feel especially good?

What does the "good feeling" feel like?

Body Scan Exercise

Every day, multiple times per day, lie down or sit comfortably. Take a few deep breaths to relax your body into the bed or chair. Start at your forehead and slowly work your way down through each part of your body, noticing how it feels. Pay attention to muscle tightness, pain, and temperature, as well as parts of your body that feel good to you. Name each sensation as you scan your body.

Step 3: Listen to your body.

Once you have gained insight into your body through Step 1 and Step 2, you will notice clearly that your body has a particular language it uses to communicate with you. This is how you become aware of your body's whispers that are trying to get your attention. These are the whispers from your body because your stress response is on.

When you find yourself feeling an emotion—whether it's anxiety, grief, guilt, loneliness, fear, helplessness—ask yourself these two questions:

1. *How is my body feeling right now?*

    This will tell you where you are holding this emotion in your body. For example, you might notice your heart fluttering or your stomach tightening. Maybe you will notice your head aching or shoulders tensing. Perhaps you'll recognize symptoms of your pregnancy complication intensifying. Go back to Step 2 and notice all of the sensations in your body as a result of this emotion.

2.   *What is my body telling me it needs?*

A high-risk pregnancy is a very physical experience, and the triggers for intense emotions are often physical in nature, which is why this step is critical. It doesn't matter if your mind is quiet or loud if your body is still whispering (or screaming) that it doesn't feel well. The best way to answer this question is to identify what would relieve the symptom. For example, if you are anxious and you notice your neck stiffening, ask your partner for a neck rub. Addressing the physical symptoms conveys to your body that you are safe and taken care of. When you establish that safety, your stress response turns off and the self-repair mechanism can turn on. This process also alleviates the emotional charge so you can think clearly about your next steps.

When you're able to experience your body in this way, not only do you gain tremendous clarity about what your body is telling you and what you can do to help it during pregnancy, but you also gain a strong sense of control and confidence. Becoming familiar with your body and the patterns of symptoms makes it much easier to choose which tools to use to alleviate the emotional and physical symptoms, turn on the relaxation response, and manage your pregnancy complications.

For a list of recommended tools, see Appendix B.

Tools to Elicit the Relaxation Response

A high-risk pregnancy is a physically demanding experience, with many emotional triggers residing in the body and with the expression of these emotions coming out through the body, as well. Because of this, both professionally and personally, I have found body-centered tools (versus cognitive or emotional tools) to be the most effective in managing complications by turning off the stress response. This appendix contains some of my favorite and most commonly taught somatic tools that you can try on your own.

The goal of any tool you use must be to improve the physical symptoms you are experiencing. For example, if you notice preterm contractions rise when your anxiety is high, the goal is to slow your contractions. Anxiety reduction will follow. If you notice your hips ache more when you feel down, the primary goal is to lessen the pain. Mood improvement will follow.

This is why it's important to begin with the daily habits from Appendix A and become keenly aware of your body's signals, so you know how to switch from listening to the thoughts in your head to listening to the language of your body. By monitoring and tracking your physical symptoms as a gauge of effectiveness, you will know quickly which tools are truly helping you not just feel better emotionally but also improving the health of your pregnancy.

Please remember that none of these are meant to be cures for your pregnancy complications, nor are they meant to replace medical care provided by your doctor. They are designed to activate your parasympathetic nervous system so you can turn off the stress response and turn on the self-healing system that's built into your body. The more often you can turn on this self-repair mechanism, the better your body can work to help you stay pregnant and help your baby grow and thrive.

Deep Breathing

Effective for:

preterm contractions, shortening cervix, elevated blood pressure, increased heart rate, tightness in muscles, insomnia, irritable uterus

Method:

Sit comfortably in a chair with your feet planted firmly on the ground and your hands in your lap or by your side. Close your eyes and breathe in through your nose for a count of 4 or 5. If you're close to the end of your pregnancy and can only breathe in to a count of 3, that's okay. Feel your lungs fill up with air as your chest expands. Breathe out for double what you breathed in.

Please note that this tool is not effective if you're experiencing high anxiety or panic.

Progressive Relaxation

Effective for:

preterm contractions, preterm labor, elevated blood pressure, muscle aches, pain relief, insomnia, cervical shortening, irritable uterus, tightness in muscles, fetal growth restriction, decreased blood flow to the baby, elevated blood glucose levels

Method:

Lie down as comfortably as you can. Close your eyes and take several deep breaths as you relax into the bed or sofa that you are on. Begin by bringing your attention to your forehead. Lift your eyebrows up as high as they can go, tightening the muscles in your forehead as tight as you can while breathing in. As you breathe out, relax your forehead. Next, move on to your eyelids. Squeeze them tight as you take a breath in. As you exhale, relax your eyes.

Work through every part of your body just like that: inhale while you clench the muscle, exhale while you release. When done properly this exercise should take approximately 10–15 minutes.

If you are experiencing preterm contractions, I recommend skipping the muscles in your torso, hips, and thighs and going straight from your upper back to your calves.

Please note that this exercise is not effective for managing moderate to high anxiety or panic.

For a guided audio of this exercise, visit pbres.pregnancybrainbook.com

Hum

Effective for:

muscle tension, aches and pains, headaches and migraines, hypothyroid, increased heart rate, elevated blood pressure, irritable uterus, preterm contractions, elevated blood glucose levels

Method:

Find a time when you are alone or comfortable to hum loudly. Take a deep breath in and hum until you have expelled all of the air from your lungs. To make sure you're doing this properly, put fingers on both sides of your windpipe and be sure that you feel vibrations on both sides. If you don't, you've likely stuck your head out too far. Simply bring your head back in line with your spine and try again. Doing this for several minutes can have a profound impact on your physical body.

Hold Ice

Effective for:

high anxiety or panic

Method:

For the moments when your anxiety is high and nothing else you're doing is helping, or if you feel you're on the brink of a panic attack, hold on to a piece of ice or something equally cold for as long as is comfortable. Don't have access to ice to hold? Try drinking ice water. (Don't drink anything with sugar or caffeine, including iced tea or fruit juice.) This strong sensory input acts like a short circuit to your nervous system, quieting it down quickly.

Re-Create Peace

Effective for:

preterm contractions, preterm labor, elevated blood pressure, muscle tension, muscular aches and pain,

Method:

Imagine a time when you were feeling at peace and when you were feeling your best physically. Use all five of your senses to immerse yourself into that moment in your memory. Notice what elements of that memory jump out at you as sources of calm. Is it the sound of windchimes in the breeze? The bright turquoise of the ocean? The smell of baking bread? Using your senses, select two or three of the most prominent elements and bring them into your current world. For example, if the color of the water was especially powerful, find ways to incorporate that color into your space by using a turquoise plate for a snack or burning a turquoise candle by your bedside at night.

Deep Relaxation Training

Effective for:

muscle aches and pains, headaches, migraines, preterm contractions, irritable uterus, decreased blood flow, elevated blood glucose levels, increased heart rate, elevated blood pressure, insomnia

Method:

Select one symptom that is particularly bothersome to you at this moment. For example, let's say you chose preterm contractions as worrying you and concerning you the most.

Lie down comfortably and close your eyes. Take a few deep breaths to relax your body into the bed or sofa you're on.

When you're ready, quietly say aloud, "I am completely calm."

Then focus your attention on the part of your body that's concerning you right now (for example, your uterus) and say out loud, "My uterus is calm and quiet." Then say aloud, "I am completely calm." Refocus your attention on your uterus and say out loud, "My uterus is calm." Say again aloud, "I am completely calm." Say aloud, "I am completely calm." Refocus your attention on your uterus and repeat, "My uterus is calm and quiet."

Repeat this until you feel your uterus calm and your whole body relax.

Please note this is exercise is not advised if you have recently experienced a heart attack, are diagnosed with a psychotic disorder and is not meant for young children.

Mindful Meditation

Effective for:

muscle aches and pains, headaches, migraines, preterm contractions, elevated blood pressure, increased blood glucose levels, elevated heart rate, insomnia,

Method:

Lie down or sit in a comfortable position. Close your eyes and put your hands on your belly. Breathe in through your nose as deeply as you can; on the exhale, say out loud, "We are okay." Once you've exhaled all of the air from your lungs, take another deep breath in and repeat.

It's okay to have other thoughts floating through your mind. The goal is not total mental emptiness. Allow the thoughts to come as they do, but keep your focus on your hands and your body and how they feel.

Chapter Notes

Introduction

1. Cousins, *Anatomy of an Illness.*
2. Janke, "The Effect."
3. Turner, *Radical Remission.*
4. Meadows, *The Other Side.*
5. Benson and Klipper, *The Relaxation Response*; Cousins, *Head First.*
6. Wadhwa, Culhane, Rauh, Barve, Hogan, Sandman, Hotel, et al., "Stress, Infection"; Lilliecreutz, Larén, Sydsjö, and Josefsson, "Effect of Maternal."
7. Northrup, *Women's Bodies.*
8. Andrews, *Stress Solutions.*
9. Lynch, Sundaram, Maisog, Sweeney, and Louis, "Preconception Stress."
10. Lipton, *The Biology.*; Yanowitz, "Impact."
11. Coussons-Read, "The Psychoneuroimmunology."
12. Smith and Nicholzon, "Corticotrophin."
13. Fischer, Heusser, and Schobel, "The Autonomic"; Vianna, Moisés, Dornfeld, and Chies, "Distress Conditions"; Schobel, Fischer, Heuszer, Geiger, and Schmieder, "Preeclampsia—A State."
14. Christian, "Psychoneuroimmunology."
15. Dunkel-Schetter, "Stress Processes."

pregnancy brain.

16. de Paz, Sanchez, Huaman, Chang, Pacora, Garcia, Ananth, Qiu, and Williams, "Risk of Placental."
17. Benson, Beary, and Carol, "The Relaxation Response."
18. Benson and Proctor, *Relaxation Revolution.*
19. Benson and Klipper, *The Relaxation Response.*
20. Frederiksen, Farver-Vestergaard, Skovgård, Ingerslev, and Zachariae, "Efficacy."
21. Benson, "The Nocebo Effect."
22. Benson and Klipper, *The Relaxation Response.*
23. Janke, "The Effect."
24. Chuang, Lin, Cheng, Chen, Wu, and Chang, "The Effectiveness"; Savitz and Schetter, "Behavioral and Psychosocial"; Vaziri, Asadi, Doracvandi, and Sayadi, "Relaxation Therapy."
25. Ryle, *The Concept of Mind.*
26. Marchant, *Cure,* p. 256.
27. Benson and Klipper, *The Relaxation Response.*
28. Rankin, *Mind over Medicine.*

Chapter 1

1. Beecher, "The Powerful Placebo."
2. Brody and Body, *The Placebo Response.*
3. Lipton, *The Biology of Belief.*
4. Cousins, *Head First.*
5. Deckro, Domar, and Deckro, "Clinical Application."
6. Cousins, *Head First,* p. 281.

Chapter 2

1. Peckham, "Physician Compensation."
2. Weil, *Spontaneous Healing.*
3. Marchant, *Cure,* p. 130.
4. Brody and Brody, *The Placebo Response.*

5. Kaptchuk, et al., "Components."
6. Benedetti, et al., "When Words."
7. Kissel and Barrucand, *Placebos*.
8. Benson, "The Nocebo Effect."
9. Paarlberg, Vingerhoets, Geijn, Kurjak, and Chervenak, "Maternal Stress."
10. Hotelling, "The Nocebo Effect."
11. Janowicz-Grelewska and Sieroszewski, "Prognostic Significance."

Chapter 3

1. Andrews, *Stress Solutions*.
2. Sylvers, Lilienfeld, and LaPrairie, "Differences."
3. Rankin, *Mind over Medicine*.
4. Cousins, *Head First*.
5. McLean, Bisits, Davies, Woods, Lowry, and Smith, "A Placental Clock."
6. Butler and Behrman, *Preterm Birth*; Hobel, Dunkel-Schetter, Roesch, Castro, and Arora, "Maternal Plasma"; Silveira, et al., "Perceived Psychosocial"; Horsch, et al., "Stress Exposure"; Kurki, Hiilesmaa, Raitasalo, Mattila, and Ylikorkala, "Depression and Anxiety"; Dingfelder, "A Little-Known Epidemic."
7. Rankin, *Mind over Medicine*.

Chapter 4

1. Bradley, "Can I Grieve?"
2. Cacioppo, Hawkley, Crawford, Ernst, Burleson, Kowalewski, Malarkey, Cauter, and Berntson, "Loneliness and Health."
3. Kashan, McNamee, Abel, Pedersen, Web, Kenny, Mortensen, and Baker, "Reduced Infant Birthweight."
4. László, Li, Olsen, Vestergaard, Obel, and Cnattingius, "Maternal Bereavement."
5. László, Liu, Svensson, Wikström, Li, Olsen, Obel, Vestergaard, and Cnattingius, "Psychosocial Stress."

6. Culhane, Rauh, McCollum, Hogan, Agnew, and Wadhwa, "Maternal Stress."
7. Buckley, Sunari, Marshall, Bartrop, McKinley, and Tofler, "Physiological Correlates."
8. Schultze-Florey, Martinez-Maza, Magpantay, Crabb Breen, Irwin, Gundel, and O'Connor, "When Grief Makes."
9. Grote, Bridge, Gavin, Melville, Iyengar, and Katon, "A Meta-Analysis."
10. Hendricks, *Learning to Love.*

Chapter 5

1. Dienstbier, "Arousal."
2. Nelissen and Zeelenberg, "When Guilt Evokes."
3. Nelissen, "Guilt-Induced."
4. Dickerson, "Psychological Correlates."
5. Dickerson, Kemeny, Aziz, Kim, and Fahey, "Immunological Effects."

Chapter 6

1. Martin and Montagne, "The Last Person."
2. "Building U.S. Capacity."
3. Martin and Montagne, "The Last Person."
4. Dyche and Swiderski, "The Effect."
5. Orloff, *Second Sight.*
6. Schetter and Glynn, "Stress in Pregnancy."
7. Rankin, *Mind over Medicine.*

Chapter 7

1. Maffei, "Sleep Deprivation."
2. Qiu, Sanchez, Gelaye, Enquobahrie, Ananth, and Williams, "Maternal Sleep."
3. Chang, Pien, Duntley, and Macones, "Sleep Deprivation."

4. Kajeepeta, Sanchez, Gelaye, Qiu, Barrios, Enquobahrie, and Williams, "Sleep Duration."
5. Andrews, *Stress Solutions.*
6. Muthukrishnan, Jain, Kohli, and Batra, "Effect of Mindfulness."
7. Stahl and Goldstein, *A Mindfulness-Based Stress,* p. 1.
8. Andrews, *Stress Solutions.*

Chapter 8

1. Seligman, *Flourish.*
2. Udelman, "Hope and the Immune."
3. Wood, Perunovic, and Lee, "Positive Self-Statements."
4. Cousins, *Head First.*
5. Brody, "The Placebo Response."
6. Lipton, *The Biology of Belief.*

Chapter 9

1. Kessels, "Patients' Memory."
2. Anderson, Dodman, Kopelman, and Fleming, "Patient Information."
3. Shapiro, Boggs, Melamed, and Graham-Pole, "The Effect."
4. Mathews and MacLeod, "Cognitive Vulnerability."
5. Rangel, Camerer, and Montague, "A Framework."
6. Ottowa Personal Decisions Guide.

Chapter 10

1. Cousins, *Head First.*
2. Cousins, *Anatomy of an Illness.*
3. Cousins, "Anatomy of an Illness."
4. Dillon, Minchoff, and Baker, "Positive Emotional States."
5. Dillon and Totten, "Psychological Factors."
6. Mora-Ripoll, "Potential Health Benefits."

7. More-Ripoll, "The Therapeutic Value."
8. Dole, Savitz, Hertz-Picciotto, Siega-Riz, McMahon, and Buekens, "Maternal Stress."

Chapter 11

1. Wood and Quenby, "Exploring Pregnancy."
2. Henderson, Carson, and Redshaw, "Impact of Preterm Birth."
3. Côté-Arsenault and Mahlangu, "Impact of Perinatal."
4. Pisoni, Garofoli, Tzialla, Orcesci, Spinollo, Politi, Balottia, Manzoni, and Stronati, "Risk and Protective."
5. Côté-Arsenault, Bidlack, and Humm, "Women's Emotions."
6. Li, Wang, Wang, and Wang, "Approaches."
7. Willens, "The Impact."
8. Helbig, Kaasen, Malt, and Haugen, "Does Antenatal?"; Levine, Alderice, Grunau, and McAuliffe, "Prenatal Stress."
9. Millet, *Love in Infant Monkeys.*

Conclusion

1. Rankin, *Mind over Medicine.*

References / Additional Reading

An, Yuan, Zhuangzhuang Sun, Linan Li, Yajuan Zhang, and Hongping Ji. "Relationship between Psychological Stress and Reproductive Outcome in Women Undergoing In Vitro Fertilization Treatment: Psychological and Neurohormonal Assessment." *Journal of Assisted Reproduction and Genetics* 30, no. 1 (2013): 35–41.

Anderson, J.L., Sally Dodman, M. Kopelman, and A. Fleming. "Patient Information Recall in a Rheumatology Clinic." *Rheumatology* 18, no. 1 (1979): 18–22.

Andrews, Susan. *Stress Solutions for Pregnant Moms: How Breaking Free from Stress Can Boost Your Baby's Potential.* Twin Span Press, 2012.

Arck, Petra Clara. "Stress and Pregnancy Loss: Role of Immune Mediators, Hormones and Neurotransmitters." *American Journal of Reproductive Immunology* 46, no. 2 (2001): 117–123.

Austgulen, Rigmor, Egil Lien, Nina-Beate Liabakk, Geir Jacobsen, and Knut Jørgen Arntzen. "Increased Levels of Cytokines and Cytokine Activity Modifiers in Normal Pregnancy." *European Journal of Obstetrics & Gynecology and Reproductive Biology* 57, no. 3 (1994): 149–155.

Bastian, Brock, Jolanda Jetten, and Fabio Fasoli. "Cleansing the Soul by Hurting the Flesh: The Guilt-Reducing Effect of Pain." *Psychological Science* 22, no. 3 (2011): 334.

Baum, Andrew, and Richard Contrada, eds. *The Handbook of Stress Science: Biology, Psychology, and Health.* Springer Publishing Company, 2010.

Beddoe, Amy E., and Kathryn A. Lee. "Mind-Body Interventions during Pregnancy." *Journal of Obstetric, Gynecologic, & Neonatal Nursing* 37, no. 2 (2008): 165–175.

Beecher, Henry K. "The Powerful Placebo." *Journal of the American Medical Association* 159, no. 17 (1955): 1602–1606.

Benedetti, Fabrizio, et al. "When Words Are Painful: Unraveling the Mechanisms of the Nocebo Effect." *Neuroscience* 147:2 (2007): 260–71.

Benson, Herbert. "The Nocebo Effect: History and Physiology." *Preventive Medicine* 26, no. 5 (1997): 612–615.

Benson, Herbert, John F. Beary, and Mark P. Carol. "The Relaxation Response." *Psychiatry* 37, no. 1 (1974): 37–46.

Benson, Herbert, MD, and Miriam Z. Klipper. *The Relaxation Response.* New York: HarperCollins, 1992.

Benson, Herbert, and William Proctor. *Relaxation Revolution: The Science and Genetics of Mind Body Healing.* Simon and Schuster, 2010.

Beydoun, Hind, and Audrey F. Saftlas. "Physical and Mental Health Outcomes of Prenatal Maternal Stress in Human and Animal Studies: A Review of Recent Evidence." *Paediatric and Perinatal Epidemiology* 22, no. 5 (2008): 438–466.

Blackmore, Emma Robertson, Jan A. Moynihan, David R. Rubinow, Eva K. Pressman, Michelle Gilchrist, and Thomas G. O'Connor. "Psychiatric Symptoms and Proinflammatory Cytokines in Pregnancy." *Psychosomatic Medicine* 73, no. 8 (2011): 656.

Bradley, Mary, LCSW. "Can I Grieve if Nobody Died?" The Good Therapy Blog, GoodTherapy.org, March 14, 2016, https://www. goodtherapy.org/blog/can-i-grieve-if-nobody-died-0314165.

Braeken, Marijke AKA, Alexander Jones, Renée A. Otte, Ivan Nyklíček, and Bea RH Van den Bergh. "Potential Benefits of Mindfulness during Pregnancy on Maternal Autonomic Nervous System Function and Infant Development." *Psychophysiology* 54, no. 2 (2017): 279–288.

Brody, Howard. "The Placebo Response." *Journal of Family Practice* 49, no. 7 (2000): 649–654.

Brody, Howard, and Daralyn Brody. *The Placebo Response: How You Can Release the Body's Inner Pharmacy for Better Health.* Cliff Street Books/HarperCollins Publishers, 2000.

Buckley, Thomas, Dalia Sunari, Andrea Marshall, Roger Bartrop, Sharon McKinley, and Geoffrey Tofler. "Physiological Correlates of Bereavement and the Impact of Bereavement Interventions." *Dialogues in Clinical Neuroscience* 14, no. 2 (2012): 129.

"Building U.S. Capacity to Review and Prevent Maternal Deaths," CDC Foundation, https://www.cdcfoundation.org/building-us-capacity-review-and-prevent-maternal-deaths.

Burke-Galloway, Linda. *The Smart Mother's Guide to a Better Pregnancy: How to Minimize Risks, Avoid Complications, and Have a Healthy Baby.* Red Flags Publishing, 2008.

Butler, Adrienne Stith, and Richard E. Behrman, eds. *Preterm Birth: Causes, Consequences, and Prevention.* National Academies Press, 2007.

Cacioppo, John T., Louise C. Hawkley, Elizabeth Crawford, John M. Ernst, Mary H. Burleson, Ray B. Kowalewski, William B. Malarkey, Eve Van Cauter, and Gary G. Berntson, "Loneliness and Health: Potential Mechanisms." *Psychosomatic Medicine* 64:3 (2002): 407–17.

Cardwell, MS. "Stress: Pregnancy Considerations." *Obstetrical & Gynecological Survey* 68, 2 (2013): 119–2.

Chang, Jen Jen, Grace W. Pien, Stephen P. Duntley, and George A. Macones. "Sleep Deprivation during Pregnancy and Maternal and Fetal Outcomes: Is there a Relationship?" *Sleep Medicine Reviews* 14, no. 2 (2010): 107–114.

Chen, Chong. *Psychology for Pregnancy: How Your Mental Health during Pregnancy Programs Your Baby's Developing Brain.* Brain & Life Publishing, 2017.

Christian, Lisa M. "Psychoneuroimmunology in Pregnancy: Immune Pathways Linking Stress with Maternal Health, Adverse Birth Outcomes, and Fetal Development." *Neuroscience & Biobehavioral Reviews* 36, no. 1 (2012): 350–361.

Christian, Lisa M. "Physiological Reactivity to Psychological Stress in Human Pregnancy: Current Knowledge and Future Directions." *Progress in Neurobiology* 99, no. 2 (2012): 106–116.

Christian, Lisa M., Albert Franco, Ronald Glaser, and Jay D. Iams. "Depressive Symptoms Are Associated with Elevated Serum Proinflammatory Cytokines among Pregnant Women." *Brain, Behavior, and Immunity* 23, no. 6 (2009): 750–754.

Christian, Lisa M., Jennifer E. Graham, David A. Padgett, Ronald Glaser, and Janice K. Kiecolt-Glaser. "Stress and Wound Healing." *Neuroimmunomodulation* 13, no. 5–6 (2006): 337–346.

Chuang, Li-Lan, Li-Chan Lin, Po-Jen Cheng, Chung-Hey Chen, Shiao-Chi Wu, and Chuan-Lin Chang. "The Effectiveness of a Relaxation Training Program for Women with Preterm Labour on Pregnancy Outcomes: A controlled Clinical Trial." *International Journal of Nursing Studies* 49, no. 3 (2012): 257–264.

Cole-Lewis, Heather J., Trace S. Kershaw, Valerie A. Earnshaw, Kimberly Ann Yonkers, Haiqun Lin, and Jeannette R. Ickovics. "Pregnancy-Specific Stress, Preterm Birth, and Gestational Age among High-Risk Young Women." *Health Psychology* 33, no. 9 (2014): 1033.

Conrad, Kirk P., and Deborah F. Benyo. "Placental Cytokines and the Pathogenesis of Preeclampsia." *American Journal of Reproductive Immunology* 37, no. 3 (1997): 240–249.

Conrad, Kirk P., Theresa M. Miles, and Deborah Fairchild Benyo. "Circulating Levels of Immunoreactive Cytokines in Women with Preeclampsia." *American Journal of Reproductive Immunology* 40, no. 2 (1998): 102–111.

Copper, Rachel L., Robert L. Goldenberg, Anita Das, Nancy Elder, Melissa Swain, Gwendolyn Norman, Risa Ramsey, et al. "The Preterm Prediction Study: Maternal Stress Is Associated with Spontaneous Preterm Birth at Less Than Thirty-Five Weeks' Gestation." *American Journal of Obstetrics & Gynecology* 175, no. 5 (1996): 1286–1292.

Côté-Arsenault, Denise, Deborah Bidlack, and Ashley Humm. "Women's Emotions and Concerns during Pregnancy following Perinatal Loss." *The American Journal of Maternal/Child Nursing* 26, no. 3 (2001): 128–134.

Côté-Arsenault, Denise, and Mary-TB Dombeck. "Maternal Assignment of Fetal Personhood to a Previous Pregnancy Loss: Relationship to Anxiety in the Current Pregnancy." *Health Care for Women International* 22, no. 7 (2001): 649–665.

Côté-Arsenault, Denise, and Nomvuyo Mahlangu. "Impact of Perinatal Loss on the Subsequent Pregnancy Self: Women's Experiences." *Journal of Obstetric, Gynecologic & Neonatal Nursing* 28, no. 3 (1999): 274–282.

Côté-Arsenault, Denise, and Dianne Morrison-Beedy. "Women's Voices Reflecting Changed Expectations for Pregnancy after Perinatal Loss." *Journal of Nursing Scholarship* 33, no. 3 (2001): 239c244.

Cousins, Norman. *Anatomy of an Illness as Perceived by the Patient: Reflections on Healing and Regeneration.* WW Norton & Company, 1979.

Cousins, Norman. "Anatomy of an Illness (as Perceived by the Patient)." *New England Journal of Medicine* 295, no. 26 (1976): 1458–1463.

Cousins, Norman. *Head First: The Biology of Hope.* Penguin Books, 1989.

Coussons-Read, Mary E. "The Psychoneuroimmunology of Stress in Pregnancy." *Current Directions in Psychological Science* 21, no. 5 (2012): 323–328.

Coussons-Read, Mary E., Marci Lobel, J. Chris Carey, Marianne O. Kreither, Kimberly D'Anna, Laura Argys, Randall G. Ross, Chandra Brandt, and Stephanie Cole. "The Occurrence of Preterm Delivery Is Linked to Pregnancy-Specific Distress and Elevated Inflammatory Markers across Gestation." *Brain, Behavior, and Immunity* 26, no. 4 (2012): 650–659.

Coussons-Read, Mary E., Michele L. Okun, and Christopher D. Nettles. "Psychosocial Stress Increases Inflammatory Markers and Alters Cytokine Production across Pregnancy." *Brain, Behavior, and Immunity* 21, no. 3 (2007): 343–350.

Coussons-Read, Mary E., Michele L. Okun, Mischel P. Schmitt, and Scott Giese. "Prenatal Stress Alters Cytokine Levels in a Manner that May Endanger Human Pregnancy." *Psychosomatic Medicine* 67, no. 4 (2005): 625–631.

Culhane, Jennifer F., Virginia Rauh, Kelly Farley McCollum, Vijaya K. Hogan, Kathy Agnew, and Pathik D. Wadhwa. "Maternal Stress Is Associated with Bacterial Vaginosis in Human Pregnancy." *Maternal and Child Health Journal* 5, no. 2 (2001): 127–134.

Dayan, J., C. Creveuil, M. Herlicoviez, C. Herbel, E. Baranger, C. Savoye, and A. Thouin. "Role of Anxiety and Depression in the Onset of Spontaneous Preterm Labor." *American Journal of Epidemiology* 155, no. 4 (2002): 293–301.

de Paz, Nicole C., Sixto E. Sanchez, Luis E. Huaman, Guillermo Diez Chang, Percy N. Pacora, Pedro J. Garcia, Cande V. Ananth, Chungfang Qiu, and Michelle A. Williams. "Risk of Placental Abruption in Relation to Maternal Depressive, Anxiety and Stress Symptoms." *Journal of affective disorders* 130, no. 1 (2011): 280–284.

de Weerth, Carolina, and Jan K. Buitelaar. "Physiological Stress Reactivity in Human Pregnancy—A Review." *Neuroscience & Biobehavioral Reviews* 29, no. 2 (2005): 295–312.

Deckro, John P., A.D. Domar, and R.M. Deckro. "Clinical Application of the Relaxation Response in Women's Health." *Clinical Issues in Perinatal and Women's Health Nursing* 4, no. 2 (1993): 311–319.

Devi, Anjali. "Impact of Music on Type 2 Diabetes." *International Journal of Diabetes & Metabolic Disorders* volume 1, issue 1 (2017).

Dickerson, Sally S. "Physiological Correlates of Self-Conscious Emotions." In *The Oxford Handbook of Psychoneuroimmunology.* Oxford University Press, 2012.

Dickerson, Sally S., Margaret E. Kemeny, Najib Aziz, Kevin H. Kim, and John L. Fahey. "Immunological Effects of Induced Shame and Guilt." *Psychosomatic Medicine* 66, no. 1 (2004): 124–131.

Dienstbier, Richard A. "Arousal and Physiological Toughness: Implications for Mental and Physical Health." *Psychological Review* 96, no. 1 (1989): 84.

Dillon, K.M., B. Minchoff, and K.H. Baker."Positive Emotional States and Enhancement of the Immune System." *International Journal of Psychiatry in Medicine* 15(1) (1985–1986): 13–18.

Dillon, Kathleen M., and Mary C. Totten. "Psychological Factors, Immunocompetence, and Health of Breast-Feeding Mothers and Their Infants." *The Journal of Genetic Psychology* 150, no. 2 (1989): 155–162.

Dingfelder, Sadie F. "A Little-Known Epidemic." American Psychological Association, October 2009, http://www.apa.org/monitor/2009/10/preterm-birth.aspx.

Dole, Nancy, David A. Savitz, Irva Hertz-Picciotto, Anna Maria Siega-Riz, Michael J. McMahon, and Pierre Buekens. "Maternal Stress and Preterm Birth." *American Journal of Epidemiology* 157, no. 1 (2003): 14–24.

Domar, Alice D., and Sheila Curry Oakes. *Finding Calm for the Expectant Mom: Tools for Reducing Stress, Anxiety, and Mood Swings During Your Pregnancy.* Penguin, 2016.

Dunkel-Schetter, Christine. "Stress Processes in Pregnancy and Preterm Birth." *Current Directions in Psychological Science* 18, no. 4 (2009): 205–209.

Dunkel-Schetter, Christine. "Psychological Science on Pregnancy: Stress Processes, Biopsychosocial Models, and Emerging Research Issues." *Annual Review of Psychology* 62 (2011): 531–558.

Dunkel-Schetter, Christine, and Laura M. Glynn." Stress in Pregnancy: Empirical Evidence and Theoretical Issues to Guide Interdisciplinary Research." In *The Handbook of Stress Science Biology, Psychology and Health.* New York: Springer Publishing Company, 2011.

Dunkel-Schetter, Christine, and Lynlee Tanner. "Anxiety, Depression and Stress in Pregnancy: Implications for Mothers, Children, Research, and Practice." *Current Opinion in Psychiatry* 25, no. 2 (2012): 141.

Dyche, Lawrence, and Deborah Swiderski. "The Effect of Physician Solicitation Approaches on Ability to Identify Patient Concerns." *Journal of General Internal Medicine* 20, no. 3 (2005): 267–270.

Engel, Stephanie A. Mulherin, Hans Christian Erichsen, David A. Savitz, John Thorp, Stephen J. Chanock, and Andrew F. Olshan. "Risk of Spontaneous Preterm Birth Is Associated with Common Proinflammatory Cytokine Polymorphisms." *Epidemiology* 16, no. 4 (2005): 469–477.

Entringer, Sonja, Claudia Buss, and Pathik D. Wadhwa. "Prenatal Stress and Developmental Programming of Human Health and Disease Risk: Concepts and Integration of Empirical Findings." *Current Opinion in Endocrinology, Diabetes, and Obesity* 17, no. 6 (2010): 507.

Entringer, Sonja, Claudia Buss, Elizabeth A. Shirtcliff, Alison L. Cammack, Ilona S. Yim, Aleksandra Chicz-DeMet, Curt A. Sandman, and Pathik D. Wadhwa. "Attenuation of Maternal Psychophysiological Stress Responses and the Maternal Cortisol Awakening Response over the Course of Human Pregnancy." *Stress* 13, no. 3 (2010): 258–268.

Ertekin Pinar, Sukran, Ozlem Duran Aksoy, Gulseren Daglar, Z. Burcu Yurtsal, and Busra Cesur. "Effect of Stress Management Training on Depression, Stress and Coping Strategies in Pregnant Women: A Randomised Controlled Trial." *Journal of Psychosomatic Obstetrics & Gynecology* (2017): 1–8.

Eskenazi, Brenda, Laura Fenster, and Stephen Sidney. "A Multivariate Analysis of Risk Factors for Preeclampsia." *Journal of the American Medical Association* 266, no. 2 (1991): 237–241.

Fischer, Th., K. Heusser, and H.P. Schobel. "The Autonomic Nervous System and Pre-Eclampsia." *Zentralblatt fur Gynakologie* 121, no. 12 (1999): 603–607.

Fischer, T., H.P. Schobel, H. Frank, M. Andreae, K.T. M. Schneider, and K. Heusser. "Pregnancy-Induced Sympathetic Overactivity: A Precursor of Preeclampsia." *European Journal of Clinical Investigation* 34, no. 6 (2004): 443–448.

Frederiksen, Yoon, Ingeborg Farver-Vestergaard, Ninna Grønhøj Skovgård, Hans Jakob Ingerslev, and Robert Zachariae. "Efficacy of Psychosocial Interventions for Psychological and Pregnancy Outcomes in Infertile Women and Men: A Systematic Review and Meta-Analysis." *BMJ Open* 5, no. 1 (2015): e006592.

Friedman, Alexander, Daigo Homma, Leif G. Gibb, Ken-ichi Amemori, Samuel J. Rubin, Adam S. Hood, Michael H. Riad, and Ann M. Graybiel. "A Corticostriatal Path Targeting Striosomes Controls Decision-Making under Conflict." *Cell* 161, no. 6 (2015): 1320–1333.

Glaser, Ronald, Theodore F. Robles, John Sheridan, William B. Malarkey, and Janice K. Kiecolt-Glaser. "Mild Depressive Symptoms Are Associated with Amplified and Prolonged Inflammatory Responses after Influenza Virus Vaccination in Older Adults." *Archives of General Psychiatry* 60, no. 10 (2003): 1009–1014.

Glover, Vivette, T. G. O'connor, and Kieran O'Donnell. "Prenatal Stress and the Programming of the HPA Axis." *Neuroscience & Biobehavioral Reviews* 35, no. 1 (2010): 17–22.

Glynn, Laura M., Elysia Poggi Davis, and Curt A. Sandman. "New Insights into the Role of Perinatal HPA-Axis Dysregulation in Postpartum Depression." *Neuropeptides* 47, no. 6 (2013): 363–370.

Glynn, Laura M., Christine Dunkel Schetter, Calvin J. Hobel, and Curt A. Sandman. "Pattern of Perceived Stress and Anxiety in Pregnancy Predicts Preterm Birth." *Health Psychology* 27, no. 1 (2008): 43.

Goldenberg, Robert L., Jennifer F. Culhane, Jay D. Iams, and Roberto Romero. "Epidemiology and Causes of Preterm Birth." *The Lancet* 371, no. 9606 (2008): 75–84.

Goodin, Burel R., and Hailey W. Bulls. "Optimism and the Experience of Pain: Benefits of Seeing the Glass as Half Full." *Current Pain and Headache Reports* 17, no. 5 (2013): 329.

Grote, Nancy K., Jeffrey A. Bridge, Amelia R. Gavin, Jennifer L. Melville, Satish Iyengar, and Wayne J. Katon. "A Meta-Analysis of Depression during Pregnancy and the Risk of Preterm Birth, Low Birth Weight, and Intrauterine Growth Restriction." *Archives of General Psychiatry* 67, no. 10 (2010): 1012–1024.

Haeri, Sina, Arthur M. Baker, and Rodrigo Ruano. "Do Pregnant Women with Depression Have a Pro-Inflammatory Profile?" *Journal of Obstetrics and Gynaecology Research* 39, no. 5 (2013): 948–952.

Hartley, Catherine A., and Elizabeth A. Phelps. "Anxiety and Decision-Making." *Biological Psychiatry* 72, no. 2 (2012): 113–118.

Hedegaard, Morten, Tine Brink Henriksen, Svend Sabroe, and Niels Jørgen Secher. "Psychological Distress in Pregnancy and Preterm Delivery." *BMJ: British Medical Journal* 307, no. 6898 (1993): 234–239.

Henderson, Jane, Claire Carson, and Maggie Redshaw. "Impact of Preterm Birth on Maternal Well-Being and Women's Perceptions of Their Baby: A Population-Based Survey." *BMJ Open* 6, no. 10 (2016): e012676.

Helbig, Anne, Anne Kaasen, Ulrik Fredrik Malt, and Guttorm Haugen. "Does Antenatal Maternal Psychological Distress Affect Placental Circulation in the Third Trimester?" *PLoS ONE* 8, no. 2 (2013): e57071.

Hendricks, Gay. *Learning to Love Yourself Workbook.* Simon and Schuster, 1990.

Hetzel, Basil S., Brigid Bruer, and L.O.S. Poidevin. "A Survey of the Relation between Certain Common Antenatal Complications in Primiparae and Stressful Life Situations during Pregnancy." *Journal of Psychosomatic Research* 5, no. 3 (1961): 175–182.

Hobel, Calvin J., Christine Dunkel-Schetter, Scott C. Roesch, Lony C. Castro, and Chander P. Arora. "Maternal Plasma Corticotropin-Releasing Hormone Associated with Stress at 20 Weeks' Gestation in Pregnancies Ending in Preterm Delivery." *American Journal of Obstetrics & Gynecology* 180, no. 1 (1999): S257–S263.

Hobel, Calvin J., Amy Goldstein, and Emily S. Barrett."Psychosocial Stress and Pregnancy Outcome." *Clinical Obstetrics and Gynecology* 51, no. 2 (2008): 333–348.

Hoffman, M. Camille, Sara E. Mazzoni, Brandie D. Wagner, and Mark L. Laudenslager. "Measures of Maternal Stress and Mood in Relation to Preterm Birth." *Obstetrics and Gynecology* 127, no. 3 (2016): 545.

Horsch, Antje, et al. "Stress Exposure and Psychological Stress Responses Are Related to Glucose Concentrations During Pregnancy." *British Journal of Health Psychology* 21:3 (2016): 712–29.

Hotelling, Barbara A. "The Nocebo Effect in Childbirth Classes." *Journal of Perinatal Education* 22, no. 2 (2013): 120.

Inbar, Yoel, David A. Pizarro, Thomas Gilovich, and Dan Ariely. ""Moral Masochism: On the Connection between Guilt and Self-Punishment." *Emotion* 13, no. 1 (2013): 14.

Irwin, Michael. "Psychoneuroimmunology of Depression: Clinical Implications." *Brain, Behavior and Immunity* 16, no.1 (2002): 1–16.

Janke, Jill. "The Effect of Relaxation Therapy on Preterm Labor Outcomes." *Journal of Obstetric, Gynecologic & Neonatal Nursing* 28, no. 3 (1999): 255–263.

Janowicz-Grelewska, Anna, and Piotr Sieroszewski. "Prognostic Significance of Subchorionic Hematoma for the Course of Pregnancy." *Ginekologia Polska* 84:11 (2013).

Kajeepeta, Sandhya, Sixto E. Sanchez, Bizu Gelaye, Chunfang Qiu, Yasmin V. Barrios, Daniel A. Enquobahrie, and Michelle A. Williams. "Sleep Duration, Vital Exhaustion, and Odds of Spontaneous Preterm Birth: A Case–Control Study." *BMC Pregnancy and Childbirth* 14, no. 1 (2014): 337.

Kaplan, S.H., S. Greenfield, and J.E. Ware Jr. "Assessing the Effects of the Physical-Patient Interactions on the Outcomes of Chronic Disease." *Journal of Medical Care* 27, Supplement (1989): S110–S127.

Kaptchuk, Ted J., et al. "Components of Placebo Effect: Randomised Controlled Trial in Patients with Irritable Bowel Syndrome." *British Medical Journal* 336.7651 (2008): 999–1003.

Kessels, Roy PC. "Patients' Memory for Medical Information." *Journal of the Royal Society of Medicine* 96, no. 5 (2003): 219–222.

Khashan, Ali S., Roseanne McNamee, Kathryn M. Abel, Marianne G. Pedersen, Roger T. Webb, Louise C. Kenny, Preben Bo Mortensen, and Philip N. Baker. "Reduced Infant Birthweight Consequent upon Maternal Exposure to Severe Life Events." *Psychosomatic Medicine* 70, no. 6 (2008): 688–694.

Kiecolt-Glaser, Janice K., Phillip T. Marucha, A. M. Mercado, William B. Malarkey, and Ronald Glaser. "Slowing of Wound Healing by Psychological Stress." *The Lancet* 346, no. 8984 (1995): 1194–1196.

Killingsworth, C., C. Dunkel-Schetter, P.D. Wadhwa, and C. A. Sandman. "Personality, Stress and Pregnancy: Predicting Adverse Birth Outcomes." *Annals of Behavioral Medicine* 19 (1997): S039.

Kissel, Pierre, and Dominique Barrucand. *Placebos et Effet Placebo en Médecine.* Masson, 1964.

Kramer, Michael S., John Lydon, Louise Séguin, Lise Goulet, Susan R. Kahn, Helen McNamara, Jacques Genest, et al. "Stress Pathways to Spontaneous Preterm Birth: The Role of Stressors, Psychological Distress, and Stress Hormones." *American Journal of Epidemiology* 169, no. 11 (2009): 1319–1326.

Kurki, Tapio, Vilho Hiilesmaa, Raimo Raitasalo, Hannu Mattila, and Olavi Ylikorkala. "Depression and Anxiety in Early Pregnancy and Risk for Preeclampsia." *Obstetrics & Gynecology* 95, no. 4 (2000): 487–490.

Landsbergis, Paul A., and Maureen C. Hatch. "Psychosocial Work Stress and Pregnancy-Induced Hypertension." *Epidemiology* (1996): 346–351.

László, K.D., Jiong Li, Jørn Olsen, M. Vestergaard, C. Obel, and S. Cnattingius. "Maternal Bereavement and the Risk of Preterm Delivery: The Importance of Gestational Age and of the Precursor of Preterm Birth." *Psychological Medicine* 46, no. 6 (2016): 1163–1173.

László, Krisztina D., Xiao Qin Liu, Tobias Svensson, Anna-Karin Wikström, Jiong Li, Jørn Olsen, Carsten Obel, Mogens Vestergaard, and Sven Cnattingius. "Psychosocial Stress Related to the Loss of a Close Relative the Year before or during Pregnancy and Risk of Preeclampsia." *Hypertension* (2013): HYPERTENSIONAHA-111.

Latendresse, Gwen. "The Interaction between Chronic Stress and Pregnancy: Preterm Birth from a Biobehavioral Perspective." *Journal of Midwifery & Women's Health* 54, no. 1 (2009): 8–17.

Levine, Terri A., Fiona A. Alderdice, Ruth E. Grunau, and Fionnuala M. McAuliffe. ""Prenatal Stress and Hemodynamics in Pregnancy: A Systematic Review." *Archives of Women's Mental Health* 19, no. 5 (2016): 721–739.

Li, D., L. Liu, and R. Odouli. "Presence of Depressive Symptoms during Early Pregnancy and the Risk of Preterm Delivery: A Prospective Cohort Study." *Human Reproduction* 24, no. 1 (2008): 146–153.

Li, Tong, Ping Wang, Stephani C. Wang, and Yu-Feng Wang. "Approaches Mediating Oxytocin Regulation of the Immune System" *Frontiers in immunology* 7 (2017): 693.

Lilliecreutz, Caroline, Johanna Larén, Gunilla Sydsjö, and Ann Josefsson. "Effect of Maternal Stress during Pregnancy on the Risk for Preterm Birth." BMC Pregnancy and Childbirth 16, no. 1 (2016): 5.

Lipton, Bruce H. *The Biology of Belief 10th Anniversary Edition: Unleashing the Power of Consciousness, Matter & Miracles.* Hay House, Inc., 2015.

Lobel, Marci, Dolores Lacey Cannella, Jennifer E. Graham, Carla DeVincent, Jayne Schneider, and Bruce A. Meyer. "Pregnancy-Specific Stress, Prenatal Health Behaviors, and Birth Outcomes." *Health Psychology* 27, no. 5 (2008): 604.

Luke, Barbara. *Every Pregnant Woman's Guide to Preventing Premature Birth.* iUniverse, 2002.

Lutgendorf, Susan K., Linda Garand, Kathleen C. Buckwalter, Toni Tripp Reimer, Sue-Young Hong, and David M. Lubaroff. "Life Stress, Mood Disturbance, and Elevated Interleukin-6 in Healthy Older Women." *Journals of Gerontology Series A: Biomedical Sciences and Medical Sciences* 54, no. 9 (1999): M434–M439.

Lynch, C.D., R. Sundaram, J.M. Maisog, A.M. Sweeney, and G.M. Buck Louis, "Preconception Stress Increases the Risk of Infertility: Results from a Couple-Based Prospective Cohort study—the LIFE Study." *Human Reproduction* 29, no. 5 (2014): 1067–1075.

Maes, Michael, Willem Ombelet, Raf De Jongh, Gunter Kenis, and Eugene Bosmans. "The Inflammatory Response following Delivery Is Amplified in Women who Previously Suffered from Major Depression, Suggesting that Major Depression Is Accompanied by a Sensitization of the Inflammatory Response System." *Journal of Affective Disorders* 63, no. 1 (2001): 85–92.

Maffei, Michelle. "Sleep Deprivation Can Lead to Preterm Labor." SheKnows, March 6, 2012, http://www.sheknows. com/parenting/articles/849055/sleep-deprivation-can-lead-to-preterm-labor.

Mancuso, Roberta A., Christine Dunkel Schetter, Christine M. Rini, Scott C. Roesch, and Calvin J. Hobel. "Maternal Prenatal Anxiety and Corticotropin-Releasing Hormone Associated with Timing of Delivery." *Psychosomatic Medicine* 66, no. 5 (2004): 762–769.

Marc, Isabelle, N. Toureche, Edzard Ernst, Ellen D. Hodnett, C. Blanchet, Sylvie Dodin, and M. M. Njoya. "Mind-Body Interventions during Pregnancy for Preventing or Treating Women's Anxiety." *Cochrane Database of Systematic Reviews* 7 (2009).

Marchant, Jo. *Cure: A Journey into the Science of Mind over Body.* Broadway Books, 2016.

Martin, Nina, and Rene Montagne. "The Last Person You'd Expect to Die in Childbirth." ProPublica, May 12, 2017. https://www.propublica.org/article/die-in-childbirth-maternal-death-rate-health-care-system.

Mathews, Andrew, and Colin MacLeod. "Cognitive Vulnerability to Emotional Disorders." *Annual Review of Clinical Psychology* 1 (2005): 167–195.

Matthews, Karen A., and Judith Rodin. "Pregnancy Alters Blood Pressure Responses to Psychological and Physical Challenge." *Psychophysiology* 29, no. 2 (1992): 232–240.

McCubbin, James A., Erma J. Lawson, Susan Cox, Jeffrey J. Sherman, Jane A. Norton, and John A. Read. "Prenatal Maternal Blood Pressure Response to Stress Predicts Birth Weight and Gestational Age: A Preliminary Study." *American Journal of Obstetrics and Gynecology* 175, no. 3 (1996): 706–712.

McLean, Mark, Andrew Bisits, Joanne Davies, Russell Woods, Philip Lowry, and Roger Smith. "A Placental Clock Controlling the Length of Human Pregnancy." *Nature Medicine* 1, no. 5 (1995): 460.

Meadows, Susannah. *The Other Side of Impossible: Ordinary People Who Faced Daunting Medical Challenges and Refused to Give Up.* Random House, 2017.

Millet, Lydia. *Love in Infant Monkeys.* Soft Skull Press, 2009.

Mooy, JM, H. de Vries, PA Grootenhuis, LM Bouter, and RJ Heine. "Major Stressful Life Events in Relation to Prevalence of Undetected Type 2 Diabetes: The Hoorn Study." *Diabetes Care* 23 (2000): 197–201.

Mor, Gil, Ingrid Cardenas, Vikki Abrahams, and Seth Guller. "Inflammation and Pregnancy: The Role of the Immune System at the Implantation Site." *Annals of the New York Academy of Sciences* 1221, no. 1 (2011): 80–87.

Mora-Ripoll, Ramon. "Potential Health Benefits of Simulated Laughter: A Narrative Review of the Literature and Recommendations for Future Research." *Complementary Therapies in Medicine* 19, no. 3 (2011): 170–177.

Mora-Ripoll, Ramon. "The Therapeutic Value of Laughter in Medicine." *Alternative Therapies in Health and Medicine* 16, no. 6 (2010): 56–64.

Muthukrishnan, Shobitha, Reena Jain, Sangeeta Kohli, and Swaraj Batra. "Effect of Mindfulness Meditation on Perceived Stress Scores and Autonomic Function Tests of Pregnant Indian Women." *Journal of Clinical and Diagnostic Research* 10, no. 4 (2016): CC05.

Myers, R.E. "Maternal Anxiety and Fetal Death." In *Psychoneuroendocrinology in Reproduction.* New York: Elsevier, 1979.

Nelissen, Rob MA. "Guilt-Induced Self-Punishment as a Sign of Remorse." *Social Psychological and Personality Science* 3, no. 2 (2012): 139–144.

Nelissen, Rob, and Marcel Zeelenberg. "When Guilt Evokes Self-Punishment: Evidence for the Existence of a Dobby Effect." *Emotion* 9, no. 1 (2009): 118.

Nepomnaschy, Pablo A., Kathleen B. Welch, Daniel S. McConnell, Bobbi S. Low, Beverly I. Strassmann, and Barry G. England. "Cortisol Levels and Very Early Pregnancy Loss in Humans." *Proceedings of the National Academy of Sciences of the United States of America* 103, no. 10 (2006): 3938–3942.

Nisell, H., P. Hjemdahl, B. Linde, C. Beskow, and N.O. Lunell. "Sympathoadrenal and Cardiovascular Responses to Mental Stress in Pregnancy-Induced Hypertension." *Obstetrics and Gynecology* 68, no. 4 (1986): 531–536.

Northrup, Christiane. *Women's Bodies, Women's Wisdom: Creating Physical and Emotional Health and Healing.* Bantam, 2010.

Okun, Michele L., James F. Luther, Stephen R. Wisniewski, and Katherine L. Wisner. "Disturbed Sleep and Inflammatory Cytokines in Depressed and Nondepressed Pregnant Women: An Exploratory Analysis of Pregnancy Outcomes." *Psychosomatic Medicine* 75, no. 7 (2013): 670.

Orloff, Judith. *Second Sight.* Grand Central Publishing, 2008.

Orr, Suezanne T., Sherman A. James, and Cheryl Blackmore Prince. "Maternal Prenatal Depressive Symptoms and Spontaneous Preterm Births among African-American Women in Baltimore, Maryland." *American Journal of Epidemiology* 156, no. 9 (2002): 797–802.

Orr, Suezanne T., Jerome P. Reiter, Dan G. Blazer, and Sherman A. James. "Maternal Prenatal Pregnancy-Related Anxiety and Spontaneous Preterm Birth in Baltimore, Maryland." *Psychosomatic Medicine* 69, no. 6 (2007): 566–570.

Ottowa Personal Decisions Guide. https://decisionaid.ohri.ca/docs/das/opdg.pdf

Paarlberg, K.M., A.J.J.M. Vingerhoets, H.P. Van Geijn, A. Kurjak, and F.A. Chervenak. "Maternal Stress and Labor." *Textbook of Perinatal Medicine* (2006): 1998–2006.

Parker, Victoria J., and Alison J. Douglas. "Stress in Early Pregnancy: Maternal Neuro-Endocrine-Immune Responses and Effects." *Journal of Reproductive Immunology* 85, no. 1 (2010): 86–92.

Pearce, B.D., Jakob Grove, E.A. Bonney, N. Bliwise, D.J. Dudley, D.E. Schendel, and Poul Thorsen. "Interrelationship of Cytokines, Hypothalamic-Pituitary-Adrenal Axis Hormones, and Psychosocial Variables in the Prediction of Preterm Birth." *Gynecologic and Obstetric Investigation* 70, no. 1 (2010): 40–46.

Peckham, Carol. "Physician Compensation Report 2016." Medscape, April 1, 2016, https://www.medscape.com/features/slideshow/compensation/2016/public/overview?src=wnl_physrep_160401_mscpedit&uac=232148CZ&impID=1045700&faf=1.

Pisoni, Camilla, Francesca Garofoli, Chryssoula Tzialla, Simona Orcesi, Arsenio Spinillo, Pierluigi Politi, Umberto Balottin, Paolo Manzoni, and Mauro Stronati. "Risk and Protective Factors in Maternal–Fetal Attachment Development." *Early Human Development* 90 (2014): S45–S46.

Ponce de León, Rodolfo Gómez, L. Gómez Ponce de León, A. Coviello, and E. De Vito. "Vascular Maternal Reactivity and Neonatal Size in Normal Pregnancy." *Hypertension in Pregnancy* 20, no. 3 (2001): 243–256.

Qiu, Chunfang, Sixto E. Sanchez, Bizu Gelaye, Daniel A. Enquobahrie, Cande V. Ananth, and Michelle A. Williams. "Maternal Sleep Duration and Complaints of Vital Exhaustion during Pregnancy Is Associated with Placental Abruption." *The Journal of Maternal-Fetal & Neonatal Medicine* 28, no. 3 (2015): 350–355.

Rangel, Antonio, Colin Camerer, and P. Read Montague. "A Framework for Studying the Neurobiology of Value-Based Decision Making." *Nature Reviews Neuroscience* 9, no. 7 (2008): 545.

Rankin, Lissa. *Mind over Medicine: Scientific Proof You Can Heal Yourself.* Hay House, Inc., 2013.

Rohde, W., T. Ohkawa, K. Dobashi, K. Arai, S. Okinaga, and G. Dörner. "Acute Effects of Maternal Stress on Fetal Blood Catecholamines and Hypothalamic LH-RH Content." *Experimental and Clinical Endocrinology & Diabetes* 82, no. 06 (1983): 268–274.

Romero, Roberto, Cecilia Avila, Uma Santhanam, and Pravinkumar B. Sehgal. "Amniotic Fluid Interleukin 6 in Preterm Labor. Association with Infection." *Journal of Clinical Investigation* 85, no. 5 (1990): 1392–1400.

Romero, Roberto, Jimmy Espinoza, Luís F. Gonçalves, Juan Pedro Kusanovic, Lara A. Friel, and Jyh Kae Nien. "Inflammation in Preterm and Term Labour and Delivery" In *Seminars in Fetal and Neonatal Medicine* 11, no. 5: 317–326. Elsevier, 2006.

Romero, Roberto, Jimmy Espinoza, Juan P. Kusanovic, F. Gotsch, S. Hassan, O. Erez, T. Chaiworapongsa, and M. Mazor. "The Preterm Parturition Syndrome." *BJOG: An International Journal of Obstetrics & Gynaecology* 113, no. s3 (2006): 17–42.

Rosenbaum, Lilian. "Biofeedback-Assisted Stress Management for Insulin-Treated Diabetes Mellitus." *Biofeedback and Self-Regulation* 8, no. 4 (1983): 519–532.

Ruiz, Roberta J., Judith Fullerton, and Donald J. Dudley. "The Interrelationship of Maternal Stress, Endocrine Factors and Inflammation on Gestational Length." *Obstetrical & Gynecological Survey* 58, no. 6 (2003): 415–428.

Ryle, Gilbert. *The Concept of Mind.* Routledge, 2009.

Sandman, Curt A., Pathik D. Wadhwa, Aleksandra Chicz-DeMet, Manuel Porto, and Thomas J. Garite. "Maternal Corticotropin-Releasing Hormone and Habituation in the Human Fetus." *Developmental Psychobiology* 34, no. 3 (1999): 163–173.

Savitz, D., and C. Dunkel Schetter. "Behavioral and Psychosocial Contributors to Preterm Birth." *Preterm Birth: Causes, Consequences and Prevention* (2006): 87–123.

Schobel, Hans P., Thorsten Fischer, Karsten Heuszer, Helmut Geiger, and Roland E. Schmieder. "Preeclampsia—A State of Sympathetic Overactivity." *Obstetrical & Gynecological Survey* 52, no. 4 (1997): 211–212.

Schultze-Florey, C. R., O. Martinez-Maza, L. Magpantay, E. Crabb Breen, M.R. Irwin, H. Gundel, and M.F. O'Connor. "When Grief Makes You Sick: Bereavement Induced Systemic Inflammation Is a Question of Genotype." *Brain, Behavior, and Immunity* 26 (2012): 1066–1071.

Seligman, Martin E.P. *Flourish: A visionary New Understanding of Happiness and Well-Being.* Simon and Schuster, 2012.

Shapiro, Daniel E., Stephen R. Boggs, Barbara G. Melamed, and John Graham-Pole. "The Effect of Varied Physician Affect on Recall, Anxiety, and Perceptions in Women at Risk for Breast Cancer: An Analogue Study." *Health Psychology* 11, no. 1 (1992): 61.

Sherer, Morgan L., Caitlin K. Posillico, and Jaclyn M. Schwarz. "The Psychoneuroimmunology of Pregnancy." *Frontiers in Neuroendocrinology* (2017).

Siegel, Bernie S. *Love, Medicine and Miracles.* Random House, 1999.

Silveira, M.L., et al. "Perceived Psychosocial Stress and Glucose Intolerance among Pregnant Hispanic Women." *Diabetes & Metabolism* 40:6 (2014): 466–475.

Smith, Roger, and Richard C. Nicholson. "Corticotrophin Releasing Hormone and the Timing of Birth." *Front Biosci* 12 (2007): 912–918.

Stahl, Bob, and Elisha Goldstein. *A Mindfulness-Based Stress Reduction Workbook.* New Harbinger Publications, 2010.

Steer, Robert A., Theresa O. Scholl, Mary L. Hediger, and Richard L. Fischer. "Self-Reported Depression and Negative Pregnancy Outcomes." *Journal of Clinical Epidemiology* 45, no. 10 (1992): 1093–1099.

Steptoe, Andrew, et al. "Loneliness and Neuroendocrine, Cardiovascular, and Inflammatory Stress Responses in Middle-Aged Men and Women." *Psychoneuroendocrinology* 29:5 (2004): 593–611.

Sylvers, Patrick, Scott O. Lilienfeld, and Jamie L. LaPrairie. "Differences between Trait Fear and Trait Anxiety: Implications for Psychopathology." *Clinical Psychology Review* 31, no. 1 (2011): 122–137.

Takiuti, N.H., S. Kahhale, and M. Zugaib. "Stress-Related Preeclampsia: An Evolutionary Maladaptation in Exaggerated Stress during Pregnancy?" *Medical Hypotheses* 60, no. 3 (2003): 328–331.

Tegethoff, Marion, Naomi Greene, Jørn Olsen, Andrea H. Meyer, and Gunther Meinlschmidt. "Maternal Psychosocial Adversity during Pregnancy Is Associated with Length of Gestation and Offspring Size at Birth: Evidence from a Population-Based Cohort Study." *Psychosomatic Medicine* 72, no. 4 (2010): 419–426.

Thoma, MV, R La Marca, R Brönnimann, L Finkel, U Ehlert, and UM Nater. "The Effect of Music on the Human Stress Response." *PLoS ONE* 8, no. 8 (2013): e70156.

Thornton, Catherine A. "Immunology of Pregnancy." *Proceedings of the Nutrition Society* 69, no. 3 (2010): 357–365.

Turner Kelly A. *Radical Remission: Surviving Cancer against All Odds.* HarperCollins, 2014.

Udelman, Donna Lou. "Hope and the Immune System." *Stress and Health* 2, no. 1 (1986): 7–12.

Vassiliadis, S., A. Ranella, L. Papadimitriou, A. Makrygiannakis, and I. Athanassakis. "Serum Levels of Pro- and Anti-Inflammatory Cytokines in Non-Pregnant Women, during Pregnancy, Labour and Abortion." *Mediators of Inflammation* 7, no. 2 (1998): 69–72.

Vaziri, Farideh, Nasrin Asadi, Mona Doracvandi, and Mehrab Sayadi. "Relaxation Therapy on Fetal Outcomes in Complicated Pregnancies Suffering Sleep Disorders: A Randomized Clinical Trial." *Journal of Health Sciences and Surveillance System* 4, no. 4 (2017): 199–204.

Vianna, Priscila, Moisés E. Bauer, Dinara Dornfeld, and José Artur Bogo Chies. "Distress Conditions during Pregnancy May Lead to Pre-Eclampsia by Increasing Cortisol Levels and Altering Lymphocyte Sensitivity to Glucocorticoids." *Medical Hypotheses* 77, no. 2 (2011): 188–191.

Wadhwa, Pathik D., Jennifer F. Culhane, Virginia Rauh, Shirish S. Barve, Vijaya Hogan, Curt A. Sandman, Calvin J. Hobel, et al. "Stress, Infection and Preterm Birth: A Biobehavioural Perspective." *Paediatric and Perinatal Epidemiology* 15, no. s2 (2001): 17–29.

Wadhwa, Pathik D., Sonja Entringer, Claudia Buss, and Michael C. Lu. "The Contribution of Maternal Stress to Preterm Birth: Issues and Considerations." *Clinics in Perinatology* 38, no. 3 (2011): 351–384.

Wadhwa, Pathik D., Thomas J. Garite, Manuel Porto, Laura Glynn, Aleksandra Chicz-DeMet, Christine Dunkel-Schetter, and Curt A. Sandman. "Placental Corticotropin-Releasing Hormone (CRH), Spontaneous Preterm Birth, and Fetal Growth Restriction: A Prospective Investigation." *American Journal of Obstetrics & Gynecology* 191, no. 4 (2004): 1063–1069.

Wadhwa, Pathik D., Curt A. Sandman, Manuel Porto, Christine Dunkel-Schetter, and Thomas J. Garite. "The Association between Prenatal Stress and Infant Birth Weight and Gestational Age at Birth: A Prospective Investigation." *American Journal of Obstetrics & Gynecology* 169, no. 4 (1993): 858–865.

Wang, Yu-Feng. "Center Role of the Oxytocin-Secreting System in Neuroendocrine-Immune Network Revisited." *Journal of Clinical and Experimental Neuroimmunology* 1, no. 1 (2016): 102.

Weil, Andrew. *Spontaneous Healing: How to Discover and Embrace Your Body's Natural Ability to Maintain and Heal Yourself.* Ivy Books, 2000.

Willens, Ashley Nicole, "The Impact of Mindfulness-Based Prenatal Yoga on Maternal Attachment" (thesis, 2015), http://scholarworks.csustan.edu/handle/011235813/873.

Witt, WP, et al. "Maternal Stressful Life Events prior to Conception and the Impact on Infant Birthweight in the United States." *American Journal of Public Health* 104(S1) (2014): S81–9.

Wood, Joanne V., W.Q. Elaine Perunovic, and John W. Lee. "Positive Self-Statements: Power for Some, Peril for Others." *Psychological Science* 20, no. 7 (2009): 860–866.

Wood, Lorna, and Shiobhan Quenby. "Exploring Pregnancy following a Pre-Term Birth or Pregnancy Loss." *British Journal of Midwifery* 18, no. 6 (2010): 350–356.

Yanowitz, Toby Debra. "Impact of Psychological Stress on Obstetric and Neonatal Outcomes among Women with Preterm Premature Rupture of the Fetal Membranes (PPROM)" (PhD dissertation, University of Pittsburgh, 2009).

Zachariah, Rachel. "Social Support, Life Stress, and Anxiety as Predictors of Pregnancy Complications in Low-Income Women." *Research in Nursing & Health* 32, no. 4 (2009): 391–404.

Acknowledgments

Writing this book has been a life-changing experience that I could never have done alone. I am eternally grateful to my village near and far, who have cheered me on, supported me, and encouraged me every step of the way.

First and foremost, huge thank you to Jodi for being my coach, mentor, advisor, and the best editor any author could have. Your reassurance, encouragement, and access to your vault of knowledge kept me sane throughout the process. You are amazing.

To Jani for seeing the power of my story and helping me find the courage to share it on Delivering Miracles® and in this book. Thank you for your patience and compassion as I found my voice again.

To Angela and Jocelyn for everything you do to keep the wheels turning behind the scenes. You both go above and beyond, and your love and support for me, my family, and the work I do are palpable. This book wouldn't have been possible without you.

A very special thank you to my colleagues and friends who encouraged me and kept me on track throughout this entire book-writing process: Lily, Arianna, Adriana, Hannah, Christine, Reina, Kat, Maria, Angela, Andrea, and Katie.

My deepest gratitude to the pioneers of the field of perinatal stress and mind-body medicine during pregnancy. Without your vision, hard work, dedication, and commitment to improving the health and lives of women and families around the world, this book would not exist. Thank you to Dr. Susan Andrews, Dr. Calvin Hobel, Dr. Patik Wadhwa, Dr. Mary Coussons-Read, Dr. Chris Dunkel-Schetter, Dr. Lissa Rankin, Dr. Christine Guardino, Dr. Thomas O'Connor, Dr. Bruce Lipton, Dr. Norman Cousins, and, last but not least, Dr. Herbert Benson for the tremendous work you do for women and families like mine.

Thank you to all of the OBs and MFMs in my referral program who trust me with their patients care. And to all of my clients, thank you from the bottom of my heart for allowing me into your life, your world, and your family. I carry each of you and your little miracles in my heart daily.

I have tremendous gratitude to every doctor, nurse, lab tech, and physician's assistant whom I met along the way on this crazy journey to bringing Vihaan home. There will never be any words to fully capture how appreciative we are of each and every one of you for your care as we fought alongside Vihaan. You are forever our family.

Thank you to lifelong friends and sisters Kavita, Ekta, and Lisa for always believing in me and never letting me forget it. Your friendship means more than any words in any language can ever express. To my amazing girlfriends (and your partners!) for the delicious food, foot massages, and mani/pedis when I was on bed rest. You brought light to some of my darkest days.

To my dad, who is my rock. My success is because of you. Thank you, also, for never making vinegar eggs again. To my strong and courageous mom for being with me during the lowest of lows and highest of highs, and teaching me what it means to be a fierce mother. Also, thank you for the donuts! To my brother for the laughs and to my "bestest friend in the whole world" for your unwavering love. To the M's, you are my world. Thank you for being the best cheerleaders I could ask for. To Kayla for picking up the pieces when I couldn't hold them all in my arms.

To all of the friends and family near and far who visited, called, texted, prayed, sent flowers and gifts, and created care baskets while Vihaan and I were in the hospital and since he came home. There are hundreds of you, but know that each and every one of you has a special place in my heart. I'm certain we wouldn't be here it weren't for you and your love.

To Sonil for the sacrifices you've made so that we could have the life we have today. Thank you for supporting my work, my passions, and my crazy ideas. I'm the luckiest girl in the world to have you as my husband.

Last but not least, thank you to Vihaan for your patience as I wrote this book. One day, I can't wait for you to read it and really understand the change you've inspired in this world. I am eternally grateful that you chose me to be your mom.

ABOUT THE AUTHOR

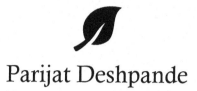

Parijat Deshpande

Parijat Deshpande, MS, is the leading high-risk pregnancy expert speaker, perinatal mind-body wellness counselor, and author who guides women to quickly and effectively release their stress during their high-risk pregnancy so they can manage their complications and give their baby a strong start to life. Her unique approach has served hundreds of women to manage pregnancy complications and reclaim a safety and trust in their bodies that they thought was eroded forever. She is also passionate about helping women heal after their baby comes home, guiding them through a gentle process that allows them to break free from the trauma without retriggering old wounds and memories. Parijat is also the host of the popular podcast Delivering Miracles®, that discusses the real, raw side of family-building including infertility, loss, high-risk pregnancy, bed rest, prematurity and healing postpartum. When she's not working with clients, speaking or recording podcast episodes, Parijat loves to hike, dance, bake and spend time by the ocean near her home, where she lives with her husband, Sonil, and their son, Vihaan. Learn more about Parijat's work and upcoming speaking engagements, as well as sign up for her newsletter, at parijatdeshpande.com.

Made in the USA
Las Vegas, NV
25 June 2022